The Bloated Belly Whisperer

THE BLOATED BELLY WHISPERER

See Results Within a Week, and
Tame Digestive Distress Once and for All

Tamara Duker Freuman, MS, RD, CDN

Recipes by Kristine Kidd

ST. MARTIN'S PRESS ⁂ NEW YORK

This book is for informational purposes only and is not intended to replace the advice of the reader's own physician or other medical professional. The author has endeavored to make sure it contains reliable and accurate information. However, research on diet and nutrition is evolving and subject to interpretation, and the conclusions presented here may differ from those found in other sources. Readers, especially those with existing health problems, should consult their physician or health-care professional before adopting any nutritional changes or taking medications/dietary supplements based on information contained in this book. The author and the publisher do not accept responsibility for any adverse effects individuals may claim to experience, whether directly or indirectly, based on information contained herein.

The patient stories in this book are composite, fictional accounts based on the experiences of many individuals. Similarities to any real person or persons are coincidental and unintentional.

THE BLOATED BELLY WHISPERER. Copyright © 2018 by Tamara Duker Freuman. All rights reserved. Printed in the United States of America. For information, address St. Martin's Press, 175 Fifth Avenue, New York, N.Y. 10010.

www.stmartins.com

Designed by Richard Oriolo

The Library of Congress Cataloging-in-Publication Data is available upon request.

ISBN 978-1-250-19523-4 (hardcover)
ISBN 978-1-250-1-9527-2 (ebook)

Our books may be purchased in bulk for promotional, educational, or business use. Please contact your local bookseller or the Macmillan Corporate and Premium Sales Department at 1-800-221-7945, extension 5442, or by email at MacmillanSpecialMarkets@macmillan.com.

First Edition: December 2018

10 9 8 7 6 5 4 3 2 1

To Max and Stella

May your bellies only ever know peace

Contents

Acknowledgments

AS THE OLD SAYING GOES, it takes a village to write the Rosetta stone of bloating. Thankfully, a genius team of gastroenterologists resides in my village, and they reviewed this book for medical accuracy. Every bloated belly I've vanquished is a credit to Eric Goldstein, M.D., whose mentorship shaped me into the practitioner I am, and whose appreciation for the role of nutrition in digestive health created a model of the patient-centered gastroenterology practice. Thank you also to Yevgenia Pashinsky, M.D., for her friendship and showing the world what a doctor-dietitian collaboration should look like; I love playing Watson to her Sherlock to solve digestive mysteries of all flavors. Thanks also to Christina Tennyson, M.D., for generously sharing her expertise.

*   *   *

This book would not exist without the foresight of my brilliant agent, Carole Bidnick, who talked me out of writing the wrong book and into writing the right book—though I take full credit for my wise decision to just shut up and do everything she tells me to. Thank you for escorting me so deftly into my career as an author and for introducing me to Kristine Kidd.

Every dietitian should be so lucky as to have a talented and creative recipe developer like Kristine, who can take a set of diet restrictions and churn out inspired recipes that deliver a wholly unrestricted culinary experience. Thank you for being such a generous adviser and collaborator.

I am beyond grateful to my editor, Jennifer Weis, for believing in this project right out of the gate and for fighting so hard to find me a home at St. Martin's Press. Thank you for your confidence, dedication, and editorial prowess. Huge thanks also to Sylvan Creekmore, whose professionalism, responsiveness, and patience made my first foray into publishing such a pleasure.

Much effort went into making sure that word of this book reached the thousands of bloated bellies for whom it was intended. For this, I am grateful to the most hands-on "A-team" of marketing and publicity I could have ever hoped for: Brant Janeway, Tracey Guest, and John Karle—as well as Associate Publisher Laura Clark. When they joined forces with my savvy brain-trust from Your Expert Nation—the incomparable Bridget Marmion, Rich Kelley, and Johanna Ramos-Boyer—I knew that this book was in the most capable hands imaginable.

Thank you to Michael Storrings for designing my book's iconic cover, and to Natalie Kueneman of Roundhouse Development for creating an online home far more fashionable than my bricks-and-mortar one, www.thebloatedbellywhisperer.com.

Finally, thank you to my husband, Alex, for your love, support, and excellent housekeeping that allowed me to neglect my earthly duties and escape to write. We joked that this book was written in "stolen moments," but I recognize that many of those moments were stolen from our family life. I promise to make up all of those moments when we grow old, retire to the South of France, and are finally free to engage in uninterrupted potty talk all day long together.

PART I

INTRODUCTION

1.

Every Unhappy Belly Is Unhappy in Its Own Way: The Many Ways to Be Bloated

I STARTED MY CAREER AS a dietitian in a gastroenterology practice, fresh out of graduate school. I was light on real-life experience with people who had digestive problems, but I arrived full of textbook knowledge about all of the conditions I thought I'd encounter in my new job. I'd done my homework and read up about how to use diet to manage diarrhea and constipation, the pain of irritable bowel syndrome (IBS), and the heartburn associated with acid reflux. I felt ready to address whatever complaints my patients would bring.

But in the three years of my dietetics education and all those months spent training in the hospital, I had never once heard of the problem that patient after patient showed up complaining about: bloating.

Bloating? What did that even mean? It wasn't a clinical condition I had ever learned about, and as far as I could tell, there was no official definition of what it was and how it should be treated. So each time patients told me they were bloated, I probed deeply to understand exactly what they meant. I asked them to describe the feeling of being bloated, what times of day it happened, what circumstances brought it on, how long it lasted, what made it better, what made it worse, whether it was painful, what it looked like, what other symptoms accompanied it. I needed to understand what this "bloating" thing was so that I could help fix it.

The more bloated patients I questioned, the more I came to understand that bloating was not a single, uniform experience that could be fixed with a one-size-fits-all solution. To some, bloating described a feeling of excessive fullness after eating—sometimes even after eating very little. To others, it described a distended belly that looked "pregnant" after eating. Some people belched when bloated; others farted. When bloating was accompanied by gas from either end, it might be painful . . . or not. And when bloating was painful, it was sometimes a pressure-type pain at the top of the stomach underneath the rib cage, a series of sharp gas pains on the sides, or a crampy pain below the belly button. Some bloating was relieved after going to the bathroom, and some wasn't. Some people woke up feeling bloated, while others found that their bloating built as the day progressed. Bloating meant so many different things.

Bloating is a symptom of something else, not a medical condition unto itself, and after spending years in my medical nutrition practice interviewing thousands of patients with digestive problems, I came to recognize distinct patterns among the different types of bloating that patients presented. As these patterns became clear to me, I became better and better at matching a patient's description of their bloating experience with its most likely underlying medical cause. I was then able to recommend tailored dietary advice that would address my patient's unique brand of bloating and collaborate with their doctor to help them get the proper diagnosis and, when appropriate, the right treatment. My bloated patients were getting better, often within days of initiating the right diet regimen.

So I started writing about bloating online in an attempt to share what I'd learned with people who might not have access to a local dietitian who was highly specialized in digestive disorders. And that's when the emails and calls started pouring in. I've heard from athletes in the Middle East battling bloating as they trained for endurance competitions and computer programmers from India who suffered tough digestive consequences when following their family's traditional vegetarian diet. Mostly, though, I heard from countless people all across America who just couldn't figure out why they were so darn bloated all the time, who felt that they'd tried everything and were desperate for a solution.

A grateful patient once remarked to me that I was like her "bloating whisperer," and my husband got a good laugh about that nickname. But it stuck. While it's certainly not a title I ever aspired to as a little girl fantasizing about what I'd be when I grew up, I embrace it nonetheless. As fate would have it, learning the secret language of bloating has become something of my calling in life, and this book is my way of sharing this knowledge with all the bloated bellies I won't have occasion to meet personally. I hope it helps you or someone you love.

Every Unhappy Belly Is Unhappy in Its Own Way

A hundred and fifty years ago, the Russian author Leo Tolstoy wrote in his famous book *Anna Karenina*: "Happy families are all alike; every unhappy family is unhappy in its own way." I think the same can be said about bellies. All happy bellies are alike; every unhappy belly is unhappy in its own way. What I mean by this is that people with happy bellies have digestive systems that function exactly as they're supposed to. Their stomachs secrete the right amount of acid to get the digestion process under way efficiently. The muscle separating their stomach from their esophagus (food pipe) prevents acid or other stomach contents from refluxing backward. The nerves that control their stomachs and abdominal wall muscles direct these muscles to stretch just the right amount after eating a meal. The pacemaker cells that control stomach emptying keep food moving along into the intestines at a normal rate. Their stomachs and small intestines have sufficient levels of enzymes to break down food into absorbable nutrients effectively. Their small intestines harbor the right number of bacteria and fully absorb the nutrients in their food. Their large intestines (colons) keep undigested fiber and waste moving along at a regular pace, resulting in bathroom patterns that are as predictable as a Swiss train schedule.

Then there's everyone else.

People with unhappy bellies have digestive systems that misbehave along any number of these dimensions. Bloating can result from dysfunction at one or more of these steps in the digestive process. The trick is to figure out the underlying cause of your bloating so that effective dietary—and, when appropriate, medical—remedies can be applied. After all, every bloated belly can be bloated in its own way.

When You Hear Hoofbeats, Look for Horses, Not Zebras

Most of my bloated patients have sought answers elsewhere before they ended up in my office. They've seen at least one doctor—and often several of them. They've consulted the internet and sometimes even seen a variety of alternative medicine practitioners. Often they've undergone many tests: colonoscopies, endoscopies, blood tests, stool tests, and ultrasounds. (All normal.) Sometimes they've also tried a variety of medications, supplements, gone gluten-free, and spent hundreds of dollars on "food sensitivity" tests, still to no avail. This lack of diagnosis and resolution despite what feels like an extensive search invariably leaves my patients with the impression that whatever is causing their problems must be pretty rare, exotic, and serious.

In reality, though, almost all of the bloated patients I see are afflicted by one of just ten reasonably common and easily diagnosable medical conditions. If your doctor or other health-care provider knows what she or he is looking for, a very detailed food and symptom history is often all it takes to narrow down the possibilities to one or two leading contenders. From there, you may be just a blood test, breath test, motility test, or diet trial away from the answers you've been looking for.

To be sure, there are plenty of rarer medical conditions that cause bloating—what we call zebras in the clinical world—that are not covered in this book. That's why books like mine aren't meant to be a substitute for personalized medical advice from a well-credentialed doctor. Some very serious medical conditions—including ovarian cancer—can first appear with a bloated, pregnant-looking belly—in that case, one that's filling with fluid. If things don't feel quite right, I encourage you to make an appointment to see a medical doctor to rule out the more serious stuff.

But the odds are still overwhelming that the medical explanation for your bloating—and the range of treatment options—is indeed contained somewhere in this book. You'll understand what I mean when you encounter that one paragraph that describes your bloating experience to a T, and you feel as though I'm talking exactly about you.

This book describes those ten most common medical causes of bloating I encounter in my clinical practice—the "horses" rather than the "zebras." Chapter 2 will help you navigate this book by introducing you to your digestive anatomy, equipping you with some vocabulary, and giving you a short quiz that will help you prioritize which chapters in parts 2 and 3 to start reading first. These chapters are grouped based on the origin of your bloating—stomach or intestines—and describe each type of bloating in great detail and its medical cause, including:

- a detailed description of what that type of bloating feels like and other symptoms with which it's typically associated;

- an explanation of the underlying cause of that type of bloating;

- a discussion of the types of tests a doctor might use to diagnose the cause;

- a review of medical treatments commonly used to treat that type of bloating;

- a review of dietary remedies that are effective for the condition; and

- stories about patients of mine who experienced that type of bloating, with details about how they were diagnosed and then treated with diet, supplements, medication, and/or lifestyle changes.

The fourth part of the book goes deeper into the specifics of the various therapeutic diets I recommend for each type of bloating, with specific food lists and meal ideas. Rather than focus on laundry lists of everything you *can't* eat, I focus more on teaching you what you *can* eat. That's why I teamed up with world-class recipe developer Kristine Kidd, who created fifty fantastic recipes for this book that are tailored to the specifications required for each therapeutic diet. Kristine spent twenty years as food editor at *Bon Appétit* magazine and is no stranger to restricted diets herself; she's got celiac disease and a garlic allergy. But when life hands a true foodie a couple of diet restrictions, she hits the kitchen and finds delicious work-arounds. In other words, don't think for a minute that you'll need to subsist on bland chicken and white rice for the rest of your life just to keep your bloating at bay!

Finally, I've included an encyclopedia of dietary supplements commonly used for digestive health, with a science-based evaluation of their effectiveness and safety. Because there is so much contradictory information on these products in circulation, I believe it's important to offer an unbiased opinion about which products may be helpful and which products may be hype. For the record, I do not sell any dietary supplements; I don't get commissions or kickbacks for referring people to supplement marketers. To avoid conflicts of interest, my clinical practice has a policy of refusing visits from pharmaceutical company representatives. If I green-light a product, it's because I've seen published evidence— or have firsthand clinical experience—that it works and that it's safe.

My intention is for you to use this book to facilitate a productive conversation with your doctor. I want to equip you with the descriptive language and relevant issues to mention during your appointment so that you can help your doctor home in on the problem most likely afflicting you. I also want to familiarize you with the diagnostic process associated with these common digestive disorders so that you won't be surprised when your doctor suggests various tests, procedures, or medications. Most important to me as a dietitian, I want to empower you with effective nutritional remedies so that you can control your own symptoms. In some cases, dietary change alone can completely control bloating. In other cases, medical therapy may be called for in addition to diet. Your doctor will help you decide on the most appropriate plan for your individual case, and your belly will offer feedback as to what's working best.

This book should not replace the advice of a doctor. I am not a doctor, and I cannot dispense medical diagnoses. Even if you recognize your brand of bloating to a T in this book, you cannot assume that the associated medical diagnosis applies to you without proper testing. Your doctor may look at other pieces of information, including family history, your personal medical history, blood test results, and any other symptoms you may be experiencing to determine whether there might be another cause of your bloating that should be investigated other than the one(s) I've suggested in this book. A good gastroenterologist is worth his or her weight in gold. Find one—and never let him or her go.

Finally, if your bloating is accompanied by any of the following symptoms, you should see a doctor promptly:

- blood in your stool
- difficulty swallowing
- recurrent vomiting
- unintentional weight loss of more than a few pounds
- nutritional deficiencies, including anemia
- sudden onset of constipation not related to a change in diet
- fever
- jaundice (yellowing of your skin and the whites of your eyes)
- a "pregnant-looking" belly that is always equally distended, even when you wake up and/or haven't eaten anything in hours (in other words, there are no circumstances under which it gets flatter)
- persistent, excessive hiccuping

Now: If you're ready to figure out how to get rid of that bloated belly of yours once and for all, then let's move on to chapter 2 so you can learn the language and take my diagnostic quiz!

2.

How to Use This Book and Diagnostic Quiz (Don't Skip This Chapter!)

IF YOU'RE READING THIS BOOK, then you've got a bloated belly in need of some answers. Your quickest path to finding them is to start reading the chapters most likely to pertain to you. To help steer you to the right ones, I've designed a quiz to help you identify the causes of bloating that are most consistent with your symptoms, and I'd recommend you start reading the chapters indicated by your quiz results. Once you recognize your brand of bloating in one of the chapters, you can skip ahead to part 4 to learn more about using fiber to manage your bloating, the therapeutic diet I recommend for your type of bloating, and what supplements may be helpful—or harmful.

Another, less direct approach would be to flip directly to the section of each chapter that describes what bloating from that condition feels like and to read each one consecutively until you find the description that feels like you're reading about yourself. Then, start reading that chapter from the beginning, in its entirety, before moving on to part 4.

If you're a fellow dietitian or other clinician using this book for continuing education, then get out your highlighter and read it start to finish. Pay special attention to the types of questions asked in the quiz below as key clues to your assessment detective work, and study the descriptions of bloating in each chapter; this will help you discern the unique characteristics of each type so you'll recognize it readily when you see it.

Know the Lingo

I use a lot of terms throughout this book to describe different parts of your digestive system and its, ahem, outputs. Let's take a moment to make sure we're all on the same page with terminology.

- I use the terms *stool, bowel movement,* and *poop* interchangeably to refer to solid waste or feces. It's the stuff that comes out of your anus.

- I use the term *defecation* interchangeably with *pooping* and *moving your bowels.*

- I use the terms *gut* and *bowel* interchangeably to refer to the entirety of your intestines—both the small intestine and the colon combined. (Purists would correctly point out that, biologically speaking, *gut* should also include the stomach, but, for our purposes, we're going to use the term more narrowly, in the way most of my patients think of it.)

- I use the terms *abdomen* and *belly* interchangeably to refer to the entire midsection of your body where the digestive organs are housed. Looking from the outside, your abdomen's borders start underneath the breastbone and end all the way down where your pubic area starts.

- I use the terms *intestinal gas, flatus,* and *farts* interchangeably to refer to the gas that comes out of your anus. Your British grandmother might have called it *wind.*

- I use the terms *abdominal distension, distended,* and *bulge/bulging* to refer to an increase in girth or circumference in your waistline, such as when your belly is protruding out from its flatter, emptier state. It's what forces you to unbutton your pants when you're bloated.

- *FOS* is a common abbreviation that some doctors use when talking among themselves; it stands for "full of stool." It describes a situation in which there is so much stool in your colon that it extends all the way back, practically right up to the junction with your small intestine. I use the terms *FOS* and *backed up* interchangeably. Do not confuse it with fructo-oligosaccharides, a type of carbohydrate that causes gas in susceptible folks as described in chapters 6 and 9 that is also sometimes referred to by this acronym.

Next, on to your anatomy. The location of your bloating and/or pain can often provide a clue as to its origin, so I've provided the diagrams on the following pages to help orient you to the organs that play a role in your digestive drama and show you where they reside. For starters, note that the abdomen is divided into four quadrants: the right upper and lower, and left upper and lower. The labels *right* and *left* refer to *your* right and left, so the labels will actually appear flipped on the diagrams (since the model is facing you). These quadrants are markers that doctors often use to describe the location of abdominal pain and discomfort.

The diagram on page 13 shows the outlines of the stomach, small intestine, and colon; they are shaded so you can see roughly where they dwell beneath external landmarks. The stomach, you may note, is quite high up—right underneath the rib cage and a bit over to your left (in the picture, it will be on the model's left side, which is on your right side, since you are facing her). The small intestine is squarely in the middle of the belly, and the colon is pretty spread out: A portion of it lives in the center of the abdomen beneath the belly button, but segments of it actually snake up and down the perimeters of your abdominal cavity, crossing over above your small intestine.

If you're feeling a bit rusty as to what each of these organs actually does, the list below offers a mini refresher. We'll be talking a lot more about all of these in later chapters, where I'll explain how they may play a role in various types of bloating.

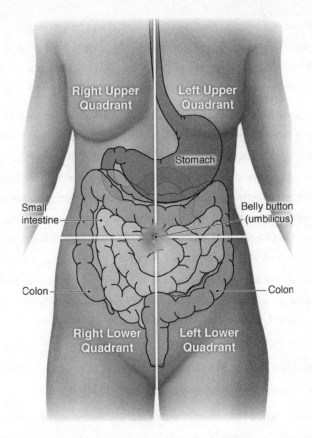

Right Upper Quadrant

Left Upper Quadrant

Stomach

Small intestine

Belly button (umbilicus)

Colon

Colon

Right Lower Quadrant

Left Lower Quadrant

- **ESOPHAGUS:** The food pipe that carries swallowed food to your stomach. It's separated from your stomach by a ringlike muscle, called a *sphincter,* that opens to let food into your stomach.

- **STOMACH:** The food storage chamber and blender that liquefies your meals so they can continue on their digestive journey. It uses acid and strong muscular contractions to work its blending magic. If you were feeling your abdomen from the outside, your stomach would be toward the top and a little to your left, just underneath the breastbone, above the belly button.

- **PYLORUS:** The muscular passageway separating your stomach from the next segment of the digestive tract, your small intestine.

- **SMALL INTESTINE:** The part of your intestines where most of digestion and nutrient absorption takes place. This is where enzymes are either delivered or manufactured to break down foods into their building blocks so they can be absorbed. If you were feeling your abdomen from the outside, much of the small intestine is located right behind and beneath your belly button, front and center.

- **COLON:** This is also called the *large intestine,* and it's where fiber and any leftover undigested food, which is now waste, arrive after leaving the small intestine. Trillions of bacteria live in the colon, and they will feast on whatever undigested food arrives here. Your colon's cells reabsorb water and some salt to help keep you hydrated, and this helps turn mushy waste into more-formed stools. If you were feeling your abdomen from the outside, the colon would cluster in the lower center portion of your abdomen beneath the belly button and then snake up the left side of your lower abdomen until just above your belly button, turning right and extending across your belly, then turning downward toward the right side of your abdomen. See the illustration on page 15 if you need help visualizing it.

- **RECTUM:** This is the six- to eight-inch, straight, final segment of your colon, where stool waits when it's ready to be eliminated.

- **ANUS:** This is the strong, ringlike (sphincter) muscle at the end of your rectum that tightens to hold in your stool and loosens when you're ready to let it pass. You can squeeze it voluntarily. In elementary school, you probably referred to your anus as your *butthole.* (In fact, you may still!)

All of these organs are pictured in the following diagram, so you can visualize how they relate to one another and where they lay underneath familiar landmarks, such as your breastbone, rib cage, and belly button.

The Bloated Belly Whisperer Quiz

I developed this quiz in collaboration with my gastroenterologist colleague Dr. Eric Goldstein as a simplified version of the detective process that goes on in our office when a new patient arrives complaining of being bloated. If you were sitting in my office, I'd pepper you with a variety of questions such as the ones following, first to help me isolate

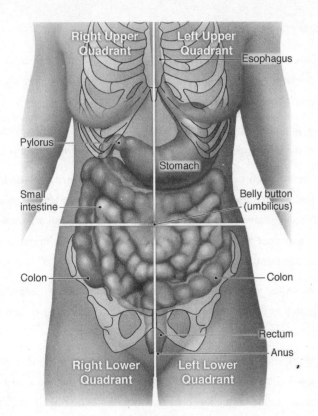

Right Upper Quadrant

Left Upper Quadrant

Esophagus

Pylorus

Stomach

Small intestine

Belly button (umbilicus)

Colon

Colon

Rectum

Anus

Right Lower Quadrant

Left Lower Quadrant

which section of your digestive tract the bloating seems to originate in, and then to narrow down the most likely one or two possibilities. While this nine-question quiz certainly doesn't cover every medical possibility under the sun, it should certainly help focus your attention on a few of the most likely possibilities.

Two types of bloating that result from malabsorption that is disease-related—celiac disease and pancreatic insufficiency—are not included in the quiz. That is because a bloated belly from either of these conditions often takes a backseat to several more troubling symptoms: copious amounts of (foul-smelling) diarrhea; stomach pain; a significant amount of unintentional weight loss; unexplained vitamin and iron deficiencies. If this sounds familiar, then call a gastroenterologist to make an appointment and flip straight to chapter 10 while his or her office has you on hold. If chapter 10 doesn't resonate with you, then check out chapter 8, on SIBO, next before trying out the quiz.

Directions for Taking the Quiz:

1. Read each question and identify the most fitting option(s) that best describe your bloating experience. For questions that allow it, you may choose more than one answer.

2. Alongside each answer, you will find one or more empty circles. **Fill in *all* of the empty circles in the row alongside the answer(s) of your choice.**

3. For any given question, **if there are no answers provided that you feel are accurate for your situation, or if you are simply unsure of an answer, *leave that question blank.*** Do not choose an answer that is the closest thing to something you experience if it is not an accurate representation of your experience.

4. When you are finished taking the quiz, count the total number of shaded boxes in each column, which are labeled A through H, and write the sum in the total box at the bottom of each column.

5. Make note of which column numbers have the highest number of shaded boxes. Look for the corresponding diagnosis and chapter/ page number in the key provided after the quiz. You should start reading the chapter/section that corresponds to the diagnosis with which you scored the most symptom matches.

6. After reading your top-ranked chapter/section, if you feel that it did not accurately describe your type of bloating, proceed to the chapter/ section where you had the second-highest number of symptom matches. (And so on.)

7. If your symptom matches score pretty evenly across multiple different types of bloating, and these include types of bloating that originate in the stomach as well as ones that originate in the intestines, you should start by reading chapter 8 on SIBO. If that description doesn't fit well, you may need to read several chapters that scored high to find the combination of diagnoses that feels most familiar. (And read the next section on common bloating combos, which may help shed some light.) Hopefully, the very detailed and differentiated descriptions of bloating I included in each chapter/section will help you narrow things down, even if your quiz results seem a little bit vague.

Consider the Common Bloating Combos

The following quiz was designed to help you identify the most likely cause of your bloating among ten of the most common possibilities. However, it's important to mention that the causes of bloating I've outlined are not mutually exclusive. In other words, it's possible—and even common—for people to have more than one reason for their bloating. This is because a single underlying medical issue can affect different parts of the digestive system. If a particular bloating description you read feels very accurate but also somewhat incomplete, you should also consider that your bloating may be the result of more than one problem. Similarly, if you follow the recommendations to address one particular type of bloating and wind up feeling a substantial improvement but still not as well controlled as you'd like, I suggest you retake the quiz with your residual symptoms in mind to see whether a second type of bloating emerges as a front-runner.

Consider some of the following examples of common medical combos that result in a double whammy of bloating and see if any of these sound familiar after reading their associated chapters:

- **GASTROPARESIS (GP, CHAPTER 3) AND CONSTIPATION (CHAPTER 7):** Sometimes problems with your digestive system's nerves will cause your entire digestive tract to operate in slow motion. The slow-to-empty stomach will produce bloating and associated symptoms in the upper GI tract, like nausea, acid reflux, or vomiting, and the slow-to-empty colon will produce bloating and associated symptoms in the lower GI tract, like farting, constipation, and crampy pain.

- **ABDOMINO-PHRENIC DYSSYNERGIA (APD, CHAPTER 3) AND CONSTIPATION (CHAPTER 7):** When the smooth muscles that govern contractions and relaxations during digestion don't coordinate properly, their dysfunction may affect muscle groups upstream in the digestive tract, downstream in the digestive tract, or both. People with APD are also prone to being constipated because of pelvic floor dysfunction (PFD), and therefore, you may experience symptoms of both: a pregnant-looking bloat after eating or drinking anything, combined with very infrequent bowel movements and lower-abdominal discomfort resulting from the inability to empty your bowels completely.

- **CELIAC DISEASE (CHAPTER 10) AND CARBOHYDRATE INTOLERANCES (CHAPTER 9):** The inflammation caused by celiac disease typically damages the fingerlike projections lining your small intestine called *villi*. Since the tips of these villi produce digestive enzymes that help you absorb certain sugars, people with newly diagnosed celiac disease may find themselves bloated not just from gluten but also from dairy foods, as the result of a temporary lactose intolerance, and/or some more sugary foods. Lactose and sugar tolerance should be restored within several months on a gluten-free diet once the gut has time to heal.

- **CONSTIPATION (CHAPTER 7) AND SIBO (CHAPTER 8):** If you've got a sluggish colon that causes chronic constipation, it's possible you could also have some slowness farther upstream in the small intestine, as well. (There are motility tests your doctor can order to determine whether this is the case.) Slow motility in the small intestine can predispose you to developing an overgrowth of bacteria there, and this may be particularly so if you've been dabbling with probiotic supplements to try to fix your constipation. If those probiotic bacteria get the chance to linger too long in the small intestine while en route to the colon, they may just take the opportunity to establish more permanent residency there.

THE BLOATED BELLY WHISPERER QUIZ

	A	B	C	D	E	F	G	H
SAMPLE QUESTION (Do not count): My bloating feels worse after chewing sugarless gum — True					●		●	●
False	O	O	O	O		O		
1. Choose one: My bloated belly is . . .								
soft	O		O	O		O	O	O
inflated like a balloon		O			O	O	O	O
solid/hard as a rock		O				O		O
2. Choose one: The location of my bloating is concentrated . . .								
broadly across the upper abdomen (above the belly button)	O	O		O	O	O	O	O
centered, right underneath the breastbone			O	O	O			
in the lower-abdominal area (underneath the belly button)						O	O	O
all over/varying locations	O	O				O	O	O

	A	B	C	D	E	F	G	H
3. Bloating onset (check up to three of the most relevant)...								
is worse/more likely with large-volume meals	O	O	O	O				
builds as day progresses; always bad/worst at night	O					O	O	
immediately after eating if I was extremely hungry at mealtime			O	O	O			
after eating anything at all	O	O		O	O			
does not seem particularly related to eating/meals					O			
4. The foods that would trigger significant bloating for me would be... (check all that apply)								
water		O			O			
large salad with olive oil and vinegar	O	O	O	O	O	O		
small plate of pasta with generous portion of red sauce		O	O		O		O	O
McDonald's-size burger and small fries	O	O		O	O			
small soft-serve frozen yogurt		O					O	O
small bowl puréed broccoli soup (no milk or cream)		O			O		O	O
5. Choose one: Do you ever wake up looking or feeling bloated?								
Yes, depending on what I ate the previous night	O					O	O	O
No		O	O	O	O	O	O	O
6. Choose one: Is your bloating associated with gas?								
Yes, belching	O		O	O	O		O	
Yes, farting				O	O		O	O
Yes, both belching and farting					O		O	
No		O						
7. In addition to bloating, I also have the following upper-digestive system issues (check all that apply):								
nausea	O		O	O			O	
vomiting	O		O					
reflux/heartburn	O		O	O	O		O	
loss of appetite	O			O		O	O	
early satiety (feeling full after eating only a small amount)	O		O	O	O			
no upper-digestive issues other than the bloating		O				O	O	O

	A	B	C	D	E	F	G	H
8. In addition to bloating, I also have the following lower-digestive system issues (check all that apply):								
infrequent bowel movements (fewer than 3 per week)		O				O	O	
feeling unable to completely evacuate my bowels when I go		O				O	O	
sticky/tar-like stools that are hard to wipe clean							O	O
hard stools, like little balls or "rabbit pellets"						O	O	
diarrhea							O	O
light-colored/orangey and loose stools							O	O
my bowel habits are not a problem	O	O	O	O	O			
9. Choose one: My bloating is associated with the following type of pain:								
no overt pain (though being bloated is generally uncomfortable)	O	O		O	O	O	O	O
burning pain toward the top of my abdomen			O	O				
sharp pain anywhere throughout my abdomen			O		O	O	O	O
crampy pain in my lower abdomen (beneath the belly button)		O			O	O	O	O
dull pain anywhere throughout my abdomen		O		O	O	O	O	O
TOTALS	A ☐	B ☐	C ☐	D ☐	E ☐	F ☐	G ☐	H ☐

Scoring the Bloated Belly Whisperer Quiz:

If you scored the most matches with column . . .	. . . your symptoms resemble this diagnosis most closely . . .	. . . so start on this chapter / page
A	Gastroparesis (GP)	chapter 3 / p. 23
B	Abdomino-phrenic dyssynergia (APD)	chapter 3 / p. 37
C	Classic indigestion	chapter 4 / p. 45
D	Functional dyspepsia (FD)	chapter 5 / p. 55
E	Aerophagia	chapter 6 / p. 69
F	Constipation	chapter 7 / p. 79
G	Small Intestinal Bacterial Overgrowth (SIBO)	chapter 8 / p. 101
H	Carbohydrate intolerances	chapter 9 / p. 118

If I did my job well, this chapter should have generated some promising leads in your quest to identify the cause of your bloating, and you've got your rank-ordered list of chapters to read. Without further ado, it's time to dive into the depths of your digestive tract and solve some mysteries!

PART II

UPPER-ABDOMINAL BLOATING THAT ORIGINATES IN THE STOMACH

3.

The "Food Baby" Twins: Gastroparesis and Dyssynergia

THE FIRST TYPES OF BLOATING we'll address have their roots in the stomach, an organ whose job it is to serve as a food storage chamber and blender. Your stomach holds the food you eat, liquefies it, and then squirts it out a little bit at a time through a tiny opening toward its bottom called the *pylorus*. The pylorus leads from the stomach into the small intestine, where the absorption of all nutrients actually happens. Your stomach's muscular walls blend food through waves of contraction and relaxation, which mix its contents with acid and enzymes to liquefy them. Then these muscular walls push the liquefied food through the pylorus to continue its path to digestion.

But when the nerves and other cells that govern your stomach's activities are not coordinating their actions properly, two distinct types of bloating can result. Both types of bloating set in quickly after eating, and they're more severe the larger the volume of the meal. Because the bloated belly in both cases results from a stomach literally filled with food, I've nicknamed this category of bloating the "food baby."

Gastroparesis (GP; Delayed Stomach Emptying)

When you eat a solid meal—or food that must be chewed, rather than a soup or a smoothie—your stomach should empty *at least* 65 percent of that meal's volume after two hours and at least 90 percent of the meal's volume after four hours. Your stomach's rate of emptying is controlled by "pacemaker" cells, which are stimulated by a number of triggers: the stretch of the stomach walls after being full from a meal, and signals from the network of nerves and hormones throughout the digestive tract. But in some cases, the stomach's pacemaker cells don't operate normally, and this can result in a delayed rate of stomach emptying called *gastroparesis* (GP).

GP affects about 2 percent of the population, and it's more common in women than in men. In many cases, the cause of GP is unknown, but it often starts in the aftermath of a viral infection; this is called *postinfectious GP*. For example, you may begin to experience symptoms of GP after recovering from a bout of food poisoning or the "stomach flu." GP is also a common side effect of both type 1 and type 2 diabetes, and in these cases, it results from damage to the digestive system's nerves as a result of chronically high blood sugar. Some medications can also induce GP, including injectable diabetes medications called *GLP-1 receptor agonists;* some examples of these include Byetta (exenatide), Victoza (liraglutide), and Trulicity (dulaglutide). GP can also result from certain types of surgery in which a major digestive system nerve is cut in a procedure called *vagotomy*.

What Bloating from GP Feels Like

Whatever the cause of your GP, its effect is the same. Bloating from GP is not typically painful, but it produces a belly that feels full and is often visibly distended. The distension is least noticeable in the morning and, in many cases, it isn't too bad after eating breakfast either. But your belly bulge grows with each subsequent meal as the day progresses, and there's usually a noticeable worsening soon after lunch. The bloating is at its absolute worst at night—particularly for those who follow the typical American custom of a relatively big dinner.

While mornings are generally the best time of day for people with GP, sometimes you might still wake up with a visibly distended belly, particularly if you've eaten a large, high-fat, and/or late dinner the night before. My patients with GP often describe feeling as if their food "just sits there" after eating, and as if they have a "brick" in their stomachs. They often experience heartburn or other symptoms of acid reflux, which can include belching or regurgitating small amounts of your acidic stomach contents when belching.

Bloating from GP is almost always accompanied by both a loss of appetite and early satiety, which means feeling very full even after eating only a small amount of food. My patients with GP rarely ever feel hungry; they often eat meals just because "I know I should" based on the time of day. With GP, you can easily go five to seven hours between meals and not feel hungry at all. Often, you'll have no appetite at all for dinner after having eaten a few small meals earlier in the day. Sometimes you may experience a strange sensation of feeling both weak from hunger but also physically too full to eat. This results from the lag time between eating food and actually absorbing its nutrients in your small intestine. In other words, blood sugar levels remain low while your slow stomach takes its time releasing its contents into your small intestine for absorption.

Nausea is very common with GP, and vomiting may occur too. This vomiting often happens at night after dinner, overnight (it wakes you from sleep), or first thing in the morning. Often, you may vomit a few hours after eating a high-fat meal (steak house dinners are a pretty common trigger) or a very bulky, high-fiber meal—like a big salad or a bucket of movie popcorn. In fact, GP is one of the few causes of bloating that is accompanied by vomiting.

Bloating from GP *is not* usually accompanied by excess flatulence (farting) or gas pain. It is typically described as uncomfortably full but not overtly painful per se.

People with GP may also experience an unintentional weight change.

In severe cases, you may have such a reduced appetite that you wind up eating very little and lose a substantial amount of weight in a short period of time. In less severe cases, you may actually gain a little bit of weight. This results from gravitating toward foods that are easier to digest and cause less bloating. For example, you may come to realize that you feel awful after eating salads—which take a long time to leave the stomach—so you start eating more foods like bread, rice, mashed potatoes, and pasta, which leave the stomach faster. This increases your daily calorie intake, and weight gain follows.

Sometimes the underlying cause of GP will also affect other parts of the digestive tract, causing slow motility not just in the stomach but also in the small intestine or the colon. In these cases, the bloating from GP that originates in the stomach may be accompanied by bloating from constipation that originates in the intestines.

Diagnosing Gastroparesis

Gastric Emptying Scan

If your doctor suspects GP based on your description of its symptoms above, then he or she will typically order a test called a *gastric emptying scan* (GES), also known as *gastric emptying scintigraphy*. This is considered the best method for diagnosis.

A gastric emptying scan is usually a two- to four-hour test conducted at a radiologist's office, and it measures how long it takes for a standardized portion of food or liquid to leave your stomach. Your stomach's emptying rate is compared against the normal emptying rate by analyzing what percentage of the food you ate remains in your stomach at regular intervals. If a larger-than-normal amount of food remains in your stomach at the end of the test, you'll be diagnosed with GP. GP is also graded into levels of severity based on what percentage of the food remains in your stomach at the end of the test; it can be mild, moderate, or severe.

When you arrive for the test, you'll be given a small meal to eat— usually oatmeal or eggs and toast. The food is mixed with a bit of radioactive material so that the radiologist can track its movement through your digestive tract by photographing your abdomen using a specialized camera. It does not use x-ray technology. Gastric emptying scans can be conducted with either liquids or solids to measure your stomach's emptying time for either of these textures. It's possible to have delayed emptying of solids but not of liquids, and even when both are delayed, generally speaking, liquids empty the stomach faster than solids.

In some cases, if your doctor suspects you may have motility problems that affect other parts of the digestive tract in addition to your stomach, he or she may order a more extensive version of this test, one which tracks the transit time of food throughout the stomach, small intestine, and colon. This test is called a *transenteric study*. A transenteric study will usually require you to be at the radiologist's office for six hours on the first day and then to come back for a quick photograph daily for the next three days.

In addition to the tests described above, there are a few additional tests that, while not specifically diagnostic for GP, may nonetheless be helpful by yielding clues to the condition's presence.

Upper-GI Series

An upper-GI series uses x-ray technology to track how liquid moves through your stomach and into the first segment of your small intestine. In this test, you'll swallow a thick liquid that contains barium, and the radiologist will monitor its flow through your digestive tract, capturing pictures along the way. The test cannot easily diagnose GP, but it is helpful in identifying whether problems with the pylorus are the cause of delayed stomach emptying in people who have already been diagnosed. For example, the test can reveal whether there's a narrowing of your pyloric opening that creates a bottleneck for food trying to pass through. This is a treatable underlying cause of GP, as doctors may be able to dilate—or stretch out—the pyloric opening. An upper-GI series is not painful, though people often complain that the barium drink is nauseating in flavor and texture; it will also likely constipate you for a day or two afterward.

Endoscopy (EGD)

Endoscopy, or EGD (a merciful abbreviation for *esophagogastroduodenoscopy*), is a test where a physician (usually a gastroenterologist) sends a tube with a camera attached to it through your mouth, down the esophagus (food pipe), and into your stomach so he or she can visualize all of these organs from the inside. The test lasts only about fifteen minutes, and it is usually done under sedation.

While EGD is not a test that doctors use to diagnose GP, sometimes they'll encounter clues that suggest the possibility of GP when scoping you for other reasons. For example, if they encounter food in your stomach that's left over from the previous night's meal, it may suggest delayed stomach emptying. This is because you're supposed to have fasted from midnight the night before for an EGD, which should give a normally functioning stomach plenty of time to empty itself. Another clue your gastroenterologist may observe during an EGD is the absence of any stomach contractions during the test. In both these cases, your doctor may recommend a follow-up gastric emptying scan.

An EGD may also reveal blockages of the pylorus that prevent food from exiting the stomach. Such blockages can be caused by scars from prior operations or ulcers that have healed, tumors, or even from bezoars, which are blobs of undigested stuff—such as food, pills, hair, or Tootsie Rolls—that clump together and can block the pylorus and prevent food from exiting the stomach.

Treating Gastroparesis

Gastroparesis treatment is generally a combination of diet change and medicine, depending on how severe the symptoms are. Because all of the medications for GP have potential side effects, your doctor may suggest that you try managing your symptoms through diet change first. There are endoscopic and surgical remedies as well.

Medical Treatment for Gastroparesis

The primary medical treatments for GP are medications called *prokinetic agents*. Prokinetics work by stimulating motility in the stomach, causing it to contract more frequently so that it will empty more rapidly and alleviate the feelings of bloating, fullness, poor appetite, nausea, reflux, and/or vomiting. Examples of prokinetic medications include Reglan (metoclopramide) and Motilium (domperidone), though the latter is not licensed for use in the United States, so most patients who use this drug import it from Canada or elsewhere overseas. The antibiotics erythromycin and Zithromax (azithromycin) also have prokinetic properties. These medications are rarely a silver bullet for GP, and diet change is almost always necessary as well.

Other medications may help control the symptoms of GP, particularly nausea and vomiting, but they don't actually address the underlying cause of the condition. Antinausea drugs (also called *antiemetics*) are one such option, though their benefit should be weighed against possible side effects. Some antiemetics may be constipating and can make bloating worse for people affected by overall slow motility in both the stomach and the colon, who are already experiencing "backed-up bloating" (see chapter 7 for more on this type of bloating).

Dietary Treatment for Gastroparesis

Dietary therapy for GP is designed to help you manage your symptoms, not to cure the disease. This is because diet cannot actually speed up the rate of your stomach's contractions. But the texture, volume, fat content, and fiber content of meals can certainly influence how quickly a meal is able to clear your slow stomach and make its way to the next phase of the digestive journey.

Choose Soft, Low-Fat, Moderate-Fiber Foods Eaten in Small, Well-Spaced Meals

Think back to the image of your stomach as a blender that I described earlier in this chapter. If your stomach blender needs to liquefy a meal for it to empty, and if the blender isn't working very well—say, it can only pulse instead of purée—what type of foods are most likely to be liquefied fastest? Meat loaf or a fatty steak? A roasted beet salad or a raw kale salad? A fruit smoothie or a big bowl of fresh pineapple? A bowl of grits or a bowl of popcorn? Peanut butter or a handful of whole peanuts?

The texture of the food arriving into your stomach matters tremendously when it comes to how quickly your sluggish stomach can empty it. Therefore, the texture of the food you eat will dictate how bloated you will feel after eating it. Anything you can do to preblend your meal before swallowing it will help, as this reduces the particle size of the food in general, and the fibers in particular, so that they will be liquefied faster. Some tips I offer my patients include the following:

- Choose cooked vegetables instead of raw ones—they'll mash up more completely when you chew and break down more quickly when encountering stomach acid.

- When eating raw fruit, choose soft, ripe, skinless options with minimal seeds.

- Use soups, smoothies, and/or juices to enable you to consume larger portions of high-fiber foods, such as fruit, leafy greens, and any produce with lots of skin, texture, and seeds. These foods may be difficult to tolerate in their whole form—whether they're raw or cooked—particularly in sizable portions.

- Choose whole-grain products with more refined textures, such as cereal flakes made from whole-grain flours; instant oatmeal; whole-grain pancakes or waffles made from flour; or light/tender whole-wheat sandwich breads. The fine texture of a whole-grain flour will move along way faster than chewy, intact cooked grains like wheat berries, steel-cut oats, or whole barley.

- Include some lower-fiber, refined grains or starchy carbs in your diet if eating too many whole-grain products aggravates your bloating; these include white rice, skinless potatoes, pasta, and white breads.

- Choose puréed forms of beans, such as hummus or fat-free refried beans, rather than whole, skin-on beans.

- Choose peanut butter or other nut butters instead of whole nuts or trail mixes.

- Seek out soft, moist, low-fat forms of protein, such as eggs, fish, shellfish, tofu, low-fat dairy, and poultry instead of fattier, chewier proteins, such as steaks, ribs, lamb, or anything fried.

- Cut your food small and chew it exceptionally well.

Chapter 12 offers a detailed, extensive discussion of the GI Gentle diet designed to manage bloating from GP, including lists of the best-textured foods by food group and the most problematically textured foods by food group. It also contains meal ideas and recipes. Flip ahead after finishing this chapter for more practical advice about which foods to focus on as your diet staples and which ones may give you trouble.

In addition to the texture of your food, the amount of food you eat in a sitting will make a difference in how bloated you feel with GP. Small meals eaten four to five times per day will feel better than three square meals per day. While the old-school advice is that people with GP should eat six to eight meals per day, I've never once met a patient with GP who could comfortably tolerate more than five mini meals per day; four is more common among the patients I've worked with. That's because most people with GP will need a solid four hours in between even modestly sized, texture-appropriate meals to allow their stomachs to empty before eating comfortably again.

Meal timing plays an important role in managing bloating from GP. If you're able to eat first thing in the morning after waking, I recommend that you do so. It will improve your ability to space meals adequately over the course of the day so that they're not piling up in a compressed time period. It's precisely this piling-up effect that contributes to your progressively worsening bloating. So if you wake at 6:30 A.M. but don't eat breakfast until 10:30 A.M., then you've missed an opportunity to squeeze in nutrition from an entire meal—particularly a meal you're most likely to tolerate, since your stomach has had a prolonged overnight period to empty. Plus, most people's appetites are generally best earlier in the day, and they dampen as the day progresses.

If you wake up feeling bloated or nauseous, or experience vomiting on most mornings, it likely means your dinner was too large and/or too late. In this case, try to stop eating for a full three to four hours before bedtime and look for ways to front-load your food intake toward the earlier part of the day, either by making meals earlier, adding a little bit more volume to earlier meals, or adding a snack before dinner so you can eat less at dinner.

SAMPLE MEAL SCHEDULE WITH GP

BREAKFAST: 6:30–8:00 A.M.

HALF LUNCH: 11:00 A.M.–12:00 P.M.

OTHER HALF LUNCH (OR SNACK): 3:00–4:00 P.M.

SMALL DINNER: 7:00–8:00 P.M.

If you need something sweet after dinner, dessert is best eaten sooner after dinner—say, by 9:00 P.M.—rather than right before bed. This will reduce the chance of experiencing acid reflux—or even vomiting—when lying down to sleep. Low-fat liquids and puréed textures will always be a better bet than solid textures. Some ideas include a cup of hot cocoa, 6 ounces of low-fat yogurt or kefir, a soft-serve fruit popsicle or small dish of sorbet, a small dish of fat-free ice cream or frozen yogurt, applesauce, fat-free pudding, and Jell-O. More ideas are listed in chapter 12.

If you still struggle with bloating, even when following a texture-modified diet with a well-spaced meal schedule, there are a few more tricks you can try. One approach that's worked well for my patients is to alternate between solid and liquid meals throughout the day. Since solid food–based meals take a bit longer to empty than a liquid meal—like a soup or smoothie—chasing the solid meal with a liquid one may allow your stomach emptying to catch up before the next solid meal comes around. If breakfast is a solid meal—say, eggs and toast—then perhaps lunch is liquid—say, a soup, and so on. Alternatively, you could start the day with a liquid meal—say, a fruit-and-protein smoothie—and follow it up with a solid lunch—say, half of a turkey sandwich with a side of steamed baby carrots. And so on.

If four meals per day still produces too much bloating, but you can't maintain a healthy weight and meet your nutritional needs on three small meals per day, then you can try moving to a three-meal-per-day model and using nutrient-fortified, clear-liquid beverages to pick up some of the nutritional slack. Many people with GP continue to drink lots of water or tea for hydration, but this can take up precious stomach real estate and crowd out space for nutritious foods. Instead, try squeezing some more nutrients into the clear liquids you're using for hydration. Some examples include protein-fortified coconut waters or coffee drinks, adding fruit-flavored protein powders to water, or sipping on a clear liquid meal replacement or protein drink (e.g., Ensure Clear, Boost Breeze, Isopure) over the course of a day. Any of these can also be frozen and made into popsicles for between-meal treats or into ice cubes to boost the nutrition of plain water.

Gastroparesis doesn't usually get better on its own—though certainly there are exceptions to every rule, and people often find that symptoms may fluctuate in terms of severity over time. For this reason, once you figure out how to choose your foods and arrange your meals on a GI Gentle diet in a manner that keeps you feeling well, you should expect to adopt this pattern of eating for the long term.

Keep Your Blood Sugar Under Control if You Have Diabetes

Having extremely high blood sugar levels, or hyperglycemia, can slow stomach emptying in people with either type 1 or type 2 diabetes. An acute episode of hyperglycemia—like when your blood sugar spikes to 200 milligrams per deciliter (mg/dL) or higher—is enough to slow down stomach emptying. (By way of comparison, a normal blood sugar level measured one hour after eating is 155 milligrams per deciliter; measured two hours after eating is 140 milligrams per deciliter.) These acute blood sugar spikes can happen as the result of forgetting to take your diabetes medications or taking an improper dose. But even when you get your medications right, hyperglycemia can result from consuming a relatively large portion of sugar and/or starches in a single sitting—like drinking juice or soda, eating cakes or cookies at a party, attacking your kids' Halloween candy haul one night when they're asleep, or eating a high-carb/high-sugar Thanksgiving meal with sweet tea, bread rolls, mashed potatoes, stuffing, cranberry sauce, and pecan pie. If you're prone to rapid blood sugar spikes, it may be helpful to consume protein- and fat-containing foods along with carbohydrate-loaded ones to help blunt their effects on your blood sugar; avoid sugar-sweetened drinks and juices; and watch your total portions of starchy foods and sweets.

Limit Use of Medically Unnecessary Pills and Supplements

People with GP should be very conservative when taking dietary supplements and pills that are not medically necessary. (For what it's worth, there are no herbal remedies or dietary supplements that speed up stomach emptying anyway.) This is because pills have coatings that can take a very long time to break down in the stomach. "Slow-release" medications can be particularly problematic, as their coatings are deliberately designed to resist breakdown in acidic stomach conditions. Many of these slow-to-dissolve pills can create a traffic bottleneck at the pylorus, delaying stomach emptying even further. People with GP are also at higher risk for an unusual type of obstruction called a *pharmacobezoar*, which is essentially a large mass of undigested pills clumping together and blocking the pylorus so that nothing can pass through into the intestine at all. This results in a backup that causes severe vomiting and often requires hospitalization to resolve.

If you have GP but must take vitamins or other dietary supplements for a legitimate medical reason, seek out liquids, chewables, gummies, sublingual tablets, or powders that dissolve in water whenever available. Often, children's versions of vitamins make fine substitutes. One way to boost nutrient intake without pills is to seek out vitamin-and-mineral-fortified breakfast foods, such as moderate- to low-fiber cereals (Cheerios, Corn Flakes, Kix, Chex, Crispix, and Rice Krispies) or instant oatmeal, farina, or grits. Be aware that organic versions of these breakfast foods tend not to be fortified with extra vitamins and minerals.

Surgical Treatments for Gastroparesis

Surgical treatment for GP is pretty uncommon, and it is generally reserved for severe cases in which you can't maintain a minimally healthy body weight through food and fortified drinks, even with the help of medication. There are a few options that your doctor may consider, and these include implanting a gastric neurostimulator device to encourage more regular stomach contractions; a jejunostomy, in which a feeding tube is placed directly into the intestine so you can bypass the stomach; having the pylorus stretched out (dilated) or removed entirely to reduce any bottlenecks preventing the stomach from emptying; and having Botox (botulinum toxin) injections—delivered via endoscopy—to help relax the pyloric sphincter so that food can flow more freely outward and onward from the stomach. Your doctor will let you know whether you're a good candidate for any of these procedures.

Sasha's Gastroparesis Story:
A Tug of War Between the Upper and Lower Digestive Tract

Sasha was a tall, athletic twenty-four-year-old woman whose only health issues were a tendency toward constipation since childhood. As a result, she tried hard to eat a very high-fiber diet—including staples such as Scandinavian bran crispbreads at breakfast, kale salads for lunch, raw carrots with hummus for a snack, and a high-fiber cereal with berries for dinner. Her high-fiber diet worked wonders to keep her regular in the bathroom, and she was moving her bowels easily and completely each day, often several times.

Following a brief illness from a stomach bug about two years ago, though, Sasha suddenly started experiencing visible bloating and feelings of nausea after meals—and increasingly, she might vomit too. She could feel completely normal for two or three weeks, but then she'd have a flare-up, during which time she might vomit after dinner, up to four times per week. Sasha started seeing a gastroenterologist, who performed both an EGD (upper endoscopy) and a colonoscopy; both turned out normal. A second gastroenterologist gave her a breath test to rule out bacterial overgrowth (see chapter 8); it was negative, but they treated her with antibiotics anyway and told her to follow a low-FODMAP diet (chapter 13). Nothing made an ounce of difference, and the bloating, nausea, and regular vomiting continued.

A third gastroenterologist diagnosed her with acid reflux and prescribed a proton-pump inhibitor (PPI) medication. The medication made a notable improvement in the severity of her nausea and frequency of vomiting, but the bloating persisted, and Sasha would still vomit about once per week after dinner. She started tracking her food and symptoms using an app and finally landed in my office.

I asked Sasha to share her food journals from the days when she experienced the worst bloating and vomiting, and a clear pattern emerged. On her bad days, she was more likely to have eaten a salad for lunch; a large/higher-fat lunch; and/or a snack within four hours of eating any meal. It didn't always matter what she ate for dinner on bad days, though larger and higher-fat dinners consistently seemed to be followed by severe bloating, nausea, and vomiting.

I was starting to suspect that Sasha's stomach might be slow to empty and that both her healthy, high-fiber lunches and her more indulgent high-fat ones were making her sluggish stomach even slower to empty. (Remember from earlier in the chapter—both fat and fiber slow down the stomach's emptying rate.) As a result, it seemed like anytime she ate an afternoon snack too soon—before lunch had a chance to clear her stomach—or anytime lunch was an extra-challenging meal for her stomach to liquefy, she'd get a "food baby" bloating attack and a wave of nausea and be at risk for vomiting.

Sasha's doctor ordered a gastric emptying scan, and it confirmed that she indeed had gastroparesis. I recommended a moderate-fiber, GI Gentle diet (chapter 12) and encouraged Sasha to part ways with raw vegetables, bran crackers, and fiber-fortified cereals. I advised three low-fat meals and one snack per day, each separated by four full hours. I encouraged Sasha to get most of her fiber from ripe, skinless fruits, softer-textured whole grains (like instant oatmeal or brown rice), and cooked veggies or vegetable soups.

Sasha was feeling much better on the GI Gentle diet in terms of abdominal bloating, nausea, and vomiting, and she could keep her symptoms controlled for weeks at a time, so long as she had some degree of control over her meals. (Travel was harder.) But soon enough, she started noticing that her old nemesis—constipation—started rearing its ugly head again. Less fiber and less roughage were alleviating her bloating and nausea but slowing her down in the bathroom; now Sasha was only having bowel movements every other day. On days she skipped, there was lots more farting. Sasha's upper GI tract and lower GI tract had competing needs, and it would be a real balancing act to figure out how to meet both of them.

Sasha's gastroenterologist and I continue to work with her to strike a comfortable balance. Her doctor put Sasha on various forms and doses of magnesium as a mild laxative (see chapters 7 and 14) until finding one that worked best, and I've been helping steer her toward super-easy-to-empty fruits and veggies for their laxative effect, such as prune juice–spiked smoothies, cooked beet salads, and veggie burgers topped with mashed avocado. As with many people dealing with a chronic GI condition, Sasha has to plan ahead to make sure she has suitable meal and snack options available to help keep her symptoms controlled.

Every once in a while, Sasha gets frustrated at her limitations and decides to just indulge in whatever she wants to eat so that she can feel "normal" again. When she does, she pays a big price in terms of bloating, nausea, and vomiting. But more often than not, she sticks to the plan and feels well. Sasha's doctor has offered her prokinetic medications that might give her more leeway with her dietary choices, but for now, Sasha says she'd rather try managing her symptoms through diet alone. If this changes in the future, Sasha knows she has a few medication options to consider trying.

Abdomino-Phrenic Dyssynergia (APD)

Dyssynergia is a general term that describes an abnormal coordination of muscle movements. This may be the result of faulty nerve signals. There are various types of dyssynergia that can affect the digestive system. One such type causes a very signature-looking type of bloating that originates in the stomach (and, technically, the small intestine as well). It is called *abdomino-phrenic dyssynergia;* we'll refer to it as APD from now on.

When you've fasted, your empty stomach is about the size of a fist. But the stomach has an amazing capacity to stretch and accommodate a very large amount of food, reaching a capacity of about a liter of volume at a time. As the fed stomach grows larger and larger inside your abdominal cavity, a muscle called the *diaphragm,* located just above the abdominal cavity, is supposed to lift up and make room for it to fit. The muscles of the abdominal wall are also supposed to relax slightly to accommodate the stretching stomach.

In the case of APD, however, the diaphragm does not lift up as it is supposed to; it may even push down into the abdominal cavity precisely as the stomach and small intestine start filling up with food and need room to expand. At the same time, the muscles that support your abdominal wall begin relaxing to an exaggerated degree. For example, you may eat just a small amount of food—say, a granola bar—and your abdominal wall muscles stretch to a degree you'd expect from eating a full

Thanksgiving meal. As a result, the stomach and small intestine, full of food, push outward against the abdominal wall, which has now relaxed in a manner so excessive that it results in significant distension outward. The result is a very pronounced, distended-looking belly that makes you look pregnant.

APD is relatively more common among people with a history of anxiety and depression. While both men and women can be affected by APD, it seems to affect young women disproportionately. Women with a history of severe anxiety, other emotional trauma, sexual abuse, and/or eating disorders may be more likely to develop APD than other people. In some cases—but not all—APD is also accompanied by dyssynergia of the pelvic floor muscles that causes constipation, difficulty passing gas (farting), and difficulty pushing out bowel movements without leaning forward or lots of pushing and straining. This is because defecation (pooping) requires pressure in the abdominal wall to generate enough force to squeeze a bowel movement out of the rectum. An overly relaxed abdominal wall cannot maintain that degree of pressure. You can read more about constipation from pelvic floor dyssynergia in chapter 7.

What Bloating from APD Feels Like

APD produces one of the most pregnant-looking types of bloating. Often, the bloating starts quite high up on the abdomen and appears puffy or swollen in the triangle underneath the rib cage, with an evenly rounded, full-looking belly underneath. Quite literally, this type of bloating can look like a "food baby." The bloated belly is *not* generally taut or stretched tight.

Another signature of APD is the occasional appearance of *guttering,* which looks like there's an indented gutter right underneath the rib cage before the swollen part of the belly puffs out. In our practice, we most commonly see this type of bloating on slim young women who show up with selfies they've taken after eating, which show very distended, pregnant-looking bellies that are at odds with their otherwise small frames.

Another unique aspect of bloating from APD is that it can be triggered even by drinking water or eating relatively small amounts of food. Anything that enters the stomach and small intestines—food, liquids, or gas—can produce bloating, though the severity of the bloating certainly depends on the volume of the meal (or beverage), as well as the properties of the food itself. Bulky, high-fiber meals will produce a more pronounced bloat than more compact, softer-textured meals. More often than not, people describe bloating from APD as uncomfortable (and emotionally distressing) rather than explicitly painful.

Diagnosing APD

If you suspect you may have APD, it will help to bring a photograph of your bloated belly at its worst to show a gastroenterologist. This is because you may not arrive bloated to your appointment, and he or she will not be able to evaluate the symptoms you're describing without a photo. While some doctors may be dismissive about generic complaints about bloating, they are far more likely to take you seriously if they see a photo of the signature pregnant-looking dyssynergic bloat.

Clinical Exam

Diagnosing APD typically involves a doctor's physical exam rather than objective criteria such as those obtained with lab tests. A doctor might examine your distended belly and notice that it feels relatively "hollow"—that is, that the belly is not full of an amount of food or gas that would match the severity of the visible distension. Your doctor might look at photographs you provide that were taken at different points of the day—upon waking, after a breakfast meal, and/or after meals later in the day. He or she may also have you drink a small amount of liquid in the office to see whether he or she can provoke the expected instant, exaggerated abdominal stretch in response to a modest amount of fluids.

Anorectal Manometry

A test that doctors use to evaluate the function of your pelvic floor muscles—the muscles that are responsible for defecation—can also be adapted to identify the presence of APD. This test is called *anorectal manometry,* and it involves a gastroenterologist placing a thin tube with a deflated balloon on the end into your rectum. The tube has sensors that measure pressure. A small amount of air is put into the tube to inflate the balloon, and you will be asked to squeeze or push or relax your muscles at various points during the test. As you do this, the machine measures whether the nerves and muscles involved in defecation are working properly.

Some doctors will add a second step to this test to help evaluate for the presence of APD; they examine how much your belly distends during the manometry test in response to inserting small amounts of air or to you bearing down as if you were trying to defecate. Some doctors might simply place a hand on your belly and feel for how much the belly distends. In our practice, the gastroenterologist actually takes out a tape measure and measures how many centimeters your abdominal girth increases during the test. (Under normal circumstances, it shouldn't distend much at all.) But this is where a doctor's clinical judgment comes in; there are currently no objective criteria of how much distension is considered normal versus abnormal. As such, it's best to seek out doctors who are more experienced with APD. They'll be more readily able to recognize it when they see it!

Treating APD

APD is not a particularly well-researched condition, and currently there is no single gold standard for treatment. At present, treatment is very personalized and generally combines multiple approaches: medication, diet changes, and physical therapy.

Medical Treatment for APD
Surfactant Medications
Because anything that fills up the stomach—including gas and swallowed air—can trigger the bloating associated with APD, using medications that break up large gas bubbles into teensy ones can reduce the severity of your belly bulge. These medications are called *surfactants.* Over-the-counter medications such as Phazyme or Gas-X (simethicone)

can be beneficial, especially if they are taken *before* eating, rather than after the fact. Less gas means less fullness, which means less distension. Surfactant medications are not absorbed into the bloodstream; rather, they remain in the digestive tract. Therefore, they are very safe and well tolerated, even with regular, long-term use. It's common for some of my patients with APD to use them before eating every meal.

Nerve-Modulating Medications

APD is a malfunction of nerve signals that causes a bloated-looking appearance. Therefore, medications that break the abnormal nerve reflex that causes excessive abdominal wall muscle relaxation can be helpful to some people. Medications in this category include those used to treat other disorders in the irritable bowel syndrome (IBS) and functional gastrointestinal condition realm (your doctor should know which they are), some antidepressants, and some neurologic drugs. While it seems paradoxical, certain muscle relaxants, like baclofen, seem to help some people as well. Because all of these medications can have side effects, it's important to discuss the risks and benefits with your doctor.

Physical Therapy and Biofeedback

Physical therapy combined with a tool called *biofeedback* (or *electromyography* [EMG]) can be used to strengthen weaker abdominal wall muscles and "reeducate" the nerves and muscles involved in digestion. In biofeedback, a trained therapist might attach sensors to the muscles of your abdomen and then guide you through a series of exercises designed to get you relaxing and contracting these muscles. As you follow the directions, the sensors will produce either a graphic display on a video monitor or an audio cue—like a particular type of beeping sound—that enables you to become more aware of a typically unconscious muscle function.

Your therapist will then instruct you to try different movements and contractions aimed at increasing muscle tension. When you achieve the desired response, you'll get a certain output on the screen or a designated audio pitch. This will let you know when you've gotten it right, and then you can practice that movement until you begin to have more control over it. Often you'll follow up with exercises at home to strengthen the muscle and help build its tension and tone.

Dietary Treatment for APD

Diet cannot cure the underlying cause of APD, which is an abnormal gut-muscle reflex, but changing your eating patterns can still help minimize the symptoms of bloating and abdominal distension.

Eat to Minimize Stomach Stretch

Adopting a soft-textured diet that involves a *grazing*-type eating pattern instead of larger, more consolidated meals, and *sipping*-type patterns rather than chugging larger volumes of liquid can minimize the stretch of the stomach and reduce the appearance of distension. Separating liquids from solid meals/snacks is also helpful.

For example, a breakfast meal may be drawn out over the course of two hours, eaten a few bites at a time with a few sips of coffee at a time, allowing the stomach time to empty as the meal progresses. You may sip on a tea or another beverage for an hour or two before the lunch meal starts, at which time you may take two hours to nibble on a soft-textured sandwich or work your way through some sushi. Perhaps there's a small, soft snack in the afternoon—a banana or yogurt—and then a break until you start working through a slow, leisurely dinner. (You can take a break halfway through the meal and come back to it rather than sit at the table for an hour or two!) Spreading out your intake in this manner should help keep hunger levels well managed so that you never feel like you're starving by the time a meal rolls around; it's impossible to control portions and eat slowly when you feel excessively hungry, and speedily eaten, large meals are certain to produce a bad case of bloating when you have APD.

If you struggle with disordered eating—both restrictive eating and binge eating—it's essential that you address your eating disorder to achieve a noticeable improvement in bloating. Many of my patients who severely restrict calories often try to fill up with large volumes of calorie-free liquids or large portions of low-calorie raw vegetables. This behavior worsens the appearance of distension from APD, as it results in a very stretched-out, full belly that takes a long time to empty. Binge eating has a similar effect, as it results in a severely overfull belly that takes hours to empty and will appear very bloated in the interim. Chronic binge eating may also have the effect of "training" the muscles of the stomach wall to loosen in response to the regularly overfull belly, resulting in an almost automatic default to exaggerated distension any time you eat anything, even regular-size meals. (Physical therapy can help strengthen and retrain these muscles, but it will only be successful if the underlying binge-eating behavior stops.)

SAMPLE MEAL SCHEDULE WITH APD

SIP COFFEE OR TEA SLOWLY OVER THE COURSE OF AN HOUR: 6:30–7:30 A.M.

STRETCH OUT YOUR BREAKFAST MEAL OVER THE COURSE OF TWO HOURS: 8:00–10:00 A.M.

SIP LIQUIDS FOR HYDRATION: 10:30 A.M.–12:00 P.M.

STRETCH OUT A SMALL LUNCH MEAL OVER THE COURSE OF AN HOUR OR TWO: 12:30–2:30 P.M.

SIP LIQUIDS FOR HYDRATION: 3:30–5:00 P.M.

SMALL, SOFT SNACK: 5:00 P.M.

STRETCH OUT A SMALL DINNER MEAL OVER THE COURSE OF AN HOUR OR TWO: 6:30–8:30 P.M.

Choosing foods from the GI Gentle diet described in the previous section on GP (and in more detail in chapter 12) is the best way to minimize stomach stretch and speed up stomach emptying—both of which help control the distended appearance of APD. Unlike the meal pattern recommended for GP, however, the eating pattern may be more fluid for APD. Flip ahead to chapter 12 after finishing this chapter for more practical advice about which foods to focus on as your diet staples and which foods to watch out for that may give you trouble.

Modifying the texture of your food and minimizing the amount of food you eat in a single sitting will often make a significant difference in the amount of bloating you experience with APD. However, since gas production in the bowel can also provoke the abdominal muscles to stretch in an exaggerated manner, some people find it helpful to limit the amount of highly fermentable (intestinal gas–producing) foods in their diets—things like beans, brussels sprouts, and fiber bars—as well.

If you have APD and sense that gas is contributing to your distended appearance, try comparing your daily diet to the lists of high-FODMAP foods contained in chapter 13. If you find that many of your go-to meal and snack staples fall into the high-FODMAP category, try replacing some of them with low-FODMAP alternatives and see if it helps.

4.

The Sour Stomach Bloat: Classic Indigestion

WHILE SOME TYPES OF BLOATING feel more chronic in nature, other types are very situational. Sour stomach bloating is one of those highly situational types of bloating; it's typically provoked when susceptible people do one of a few things:

- go too long in between meals without snacking, allowing themselves to become extremely hungry
- eat large-volume and/or high-fat meals
- drink alcohol, particularly on an empty stomach

Often, my patients struggle to identify the trigger of their sour stomach bloating, because a particular meal may go over perfectly well one day but then provoke a bloating attack when eaten on another day. Understanding the situational context that triggers an attack is often the missing piece of the puzzle.

Classic Indigestion

Indigestion isn't a medical diagnosis but rather a description of uncomfortable symptoms you may experience after eating. Bloating is one of the common symptoms that falls under the indigestion umbrella; the others are described below. Classic indigestion usually results from an underlying medical condition, such as gastritis (irritation of the stomach lining), ulcers, hiatal hernia, and/or acid reflux. Bloating that occurs in association with acid reflux or indigestion is what I've termed *sour stomach bloating*. It's this connection with acid-related problems that put the *sour* in *sour stomach bloating* and has led many marketers of antacid products to describe this type of bloating as *acid indigestion*. If there is no identifiable medical condition causing your indigestion-like symptoms, a doctor may diagnose you with *functional dyspepsia* (see chapter 5).

Indigestion is generally provoked by meals that are very large, high in fat, very spicy, and/or eaten too quickly. Drinking alcohol before such a meal may make you even more prone to experiencing indigestion.

What Bloating from Classic Indigestion Feels Like

Bloating from classic indigestion comes on immediately after eating a meal. It is typically worse after a large or high-fat meal or any meal eaten after a prolonged period of fasting—such as if you skip breakfast and don't eat your first bite until noon or after. People describe it as feeling like their bellies swell up like a balloon full of air, and quite often it's accompanied by belching. Sometimes the belching involves regurgitating small amounts of the contents of your stomach as well; most people recognize it as "throwing up a little in your mouth." The bloating is very uncomfortable in a way that feels overfull. Your entire belly may be visibly distended, but more often, the discomfort is concentrated toward the top of the stomach, underneath the breastbone.

Bloating from classic indigestion is often accompanied by acid reflux, which can make itself known through heartburn, nausea, a sore throat, or a sour/metallic taste in the mouth. If you do have heartburn, then you may actually feel pain from this type of bloating rather than just discomfort and overfullness. In rare cases, you may vomit as well.

Diagnosing Classic Indigestion

Indigestion is not a clinical diagnosis in and of itself. Still, the symptoms are so predictable that most doctors know it when they see it.

Endoscopy (EGD)

As described in chapter 3 (pages 27–28), endoscopy is a test where a gastroenterologist sends a tube with a camera attached through your mouth, down the esophagus (food pipe), and into your stomach, so he or she can see all of these organs from the inside. The test lasts only about fifteen minutes, and it is done under sedation. Your doctor may use endoscopy to see whether you have irritation in the upper stomach region (gastritis), ulcers, or evidence of acid-related damage to your stomach or esophagus. He or she may also take tissue samples to see if you are infected with bacteria called *H. pylori* that can trigger symptoms of indigestion.

Breath or Stool Testing for *H. pylori*

Sometimes instead of going straight to endoscopy, doctors will order a quick and noninvasive test of your breath or stool to detect the presence of infection with *H. pylori* bacteria. If it's positive, they may treat you with antibiotics and see how your symptoms respond before considering the relatively more invasive endoscopy. If *H. pylori* infection was the cause for your bloating and upper-abdominal discomfort, the symptoms should resolve after antibiotic treatment. However, sometimes eradicating *H. pylori* actually makes acid reflux worse in the longer term. It's a tricky dilemma, to be sure, and in our practice, we don't automatically go looking for *H. pylori* right out of the gate for precisely this reason. Instead, we often try diet modification and some basic over-the-counter remedies first before setting off in pursuit of this wily bacteria.

You'll arrive at a gastroenterologist's office after fasting for your *H.*

pylori breath test and then swallow a pill containing a compound called *urea*. During the test, which lasts only about fifteen minutes, you'll breathe into a tube so the technician can capture and analyze samples of the gases in your breath. If you're infected with *H. pylori,* then your exhaled breath will contain all the clues needed to make the diagnosis. Blood testing for *H. pylori* has fallen out of favor because it can't distinguish between an active infection and a past infection that has since been resolved.

Treating Classic Indigestion

Medical Treatment for Classic Indigestion

A variety of both over-the-counter and prescription medications are beneficial in managing bloating from indigestion.

Antacids

Antacid products are available over the counter, and they offer fast-acting but short-lived relief from sour stomach bloating. These products work by neutralizing stomach acid and helping to trigger belching, which can relieve some of the gas pressure that contributes to bloating. There are many options in the world of antacids. Chewable calcium carbonate tablets—such as TUMS, Rolaids, or Alka-Seltzer Heartburn Relief Chews—are among the best-known options. (They also do double duty as a calcium supplement, which is great news for women who may be concerned about bone health.) If you're a gum chewer who appreciates nostalgia, Chooz antacid gum is a calcium carbonate gum that my patients of a certain generation swear by. Liquid antacids containing magnesium hydroxide and/or aluminum hydroxide, such as Gaviscon, Maalox, and Mylanta, are also effective; the latter two products also contain a gas bubble–busting ingredient called *simethicone* for added bloating relief. If you've got kidney disease, however, magnesium-based antacids may not be your best choice.

Sodium bicarbonate (otherwise known as baking soda) is also an effective buffer for stomach acid. You can concoct a homemade antacid by mixing baking soda with water, which is safe for adults but not young children. The proper ratio would be a quarter teaspoon of baking soda per cup of water. Alternatively, Alka-Seltzer tablets combine sodium bicar-bonate with aspirin for mild pain relief. If you are allergic or sensitive to aspirin, or if you have a history of ulcers from using too many nonsteroi-dal pain-relieving medications, this may not be the best choice for you.

Another common antacid ingredient called *bismuth subsalicylate* can multitask by treating diarrhea in addition to the upper-GI symptoms of indigestion; it is marketed as Pepto-Bismol or Kaopectate. The active ingredient in these medications can turn your poop black, so don't be alarmed if things look amiss in the toilet for a day or two after taking them. You should avoid these products if you're allergic to aspirin.

H2 Blockers

A class of medicines called *H2 blockers* interfere with histamine-stimulated stomach acid production; common drugs in this category are Pepcid (famotidine) and Zantac (ranitidine). While the antacids described above begin working within minutes, H2 blockers take about thirty minutes to kick in. However, they last far longer than antacids—up to ten hours, instead of just an hour or so. These medications can be taken in advance to prevent symptoms in susceptible people—like at night before bed or in the morning before eating. Antacids can be taken at the same time as an H2 blocker to get immediate and long-lasting relief from indigestion; the antacid starts working immediately, and the H2 blocker starts working just as the antacid's effects begin to fade. Because H2 blockers have far fewer long-term side effects than another class of acid-suppressing medication called *proton-pump inhibitors* (*PPIs*), they are considered much safer for prolonged use, particularly for people who only experience occasional indigestion.

Proton-Pump Inhibitors (PPIs)

If you suffer from chronic indigestion and have been diagnosed with acid reflux disease (GERD), your doctor might prescribe a type of medi-cine called a *proton-pump inhibitor,* or PPI. The generic names of all the drugs in the class end with the suffix *-prazole.* (Brand names include Pri-losec, Nexium, Prevacid, Aciphex, and Protonix.) PPIs work by drasti-cally reducing the amount of stomach acid you produce—to a far greater degree than H2 blockers. They are very effective at reducing the frequency and severity of sour stomach bloating episodes, but under the right circumstances (or wrong ones, depending on how you look at it), you may continue to experience breakthrough episodes. For example, even your PPI may be no match for a large, boozy steak dinner followed by cigars.

If you haven't been diagnosed with GERD, then using a PPI to treat occasional sour stomach bloating would be like using a sledgehammer to swat a fly. Because these medications may be associated with more side effects than other types of acid-suppressing drugs, they would not be the ideal first-line treatment for sour stomach symptoms. PPIs also may be difficult to wean from once you start using them regularly; symptoms can get much worse for a period of time if you stop taking them cold turkey. Among other concerns, long-term use of PPIs may increase risk of osteoporosis, so it's important to supplement calcium and vitamin D if you are taking these meds for more than a few months. They may also predispose you to developing a condition called *small intestinal bacterial overgrowth* (or SIBO; see chapter 8). These risks are generally deemed acceptable for people with GERD, because they're outweighed by an important benefit: a reduced risk of developing esophageal cancer from chronic acid damage. But these risks may be less appropriate for people without GERD, who could manage their bloating symptoms perfectly well with a well-timed TUMS and some diet changes.

Dietary Treatment for Classic Indigestion

Dietary changes work wonders for people with sour stomach bloating from classic indigestion. If this is your brand of bloating, then an ounce of prevention can often spare you the need to rely on medication. The goal of your diet to prevent sour stomach bloat is to plan meals and snacks in a way that prevents your stomach from becoming either too empty *or* too full.

A too-full stomach can get you into trouble. Extra-full bellies take a long time to empty and predispose you to experiencing acid reflux during that prolonged emptying time. And if that large meal is also high in fat, it's practically begging for the muscle separating your stomach and esophagus to loosen up and allow acid to reflux back up the food pipe, adding heartburn and pain to your already miserable bloating experience.

But in my clinical experience, a too-empty stomach can be

problematic too. I've repeated this mantra to my patients thousands of times over the years: "An empty stomach is an acid stomach." One of the surest ways to trigger a sour stomach bloating attack is to go way too long in between meals. Once you finally eat, it's common to experience a digestive overreaction no matter what you've eaten, and this can present itself as bloating, belching, overfullness, sharp pains, or a general feeling of having an unsettled stomach. If your meal of choice on an empty stomach happens also to be a large salad, it may provoke even more bloating and discomfort than a softer-textured meal that requires less time and less acid to break down.

Eat Small Meals or Substantial Snacks Every Three Hours

The best way to prevent extremes in emptiness or fullness is to plan for a small meal or substantial snack every three to four hours. You should not go more than four hours without eating. In addition to keeping your belly calmer, eating frequently helps manage your hunger so that you're less likely to overeat portions at the next meal. As best as you are able, try to spread your intake as evenly as possible across the day's meals and snacks, so that the amount you eat at dinner is not particularly more food than what you ate at breakfast or lunch.

To achieve this, you'll want to consider what qualifies as a snack. A lone banana between lunch and dinner may not be nearly enough to help manage your hunger levels—and therefore portions—as you arrive at the dinner table. You'll also want to be sure you're not skimping on breakfast or lunch, as many of my patients are in the habit of doing. After all, if you ever arrive to a meal feeling famished from a too-light lunch or an absent breakfast, the likelihood of leaving that meal with a sour, bloated belly is high. Finally, if you've gone more than four hours without eating, consider chewing a calcium carbonate antacid right before tucking into your next meal to help neutralize some of that stomach acid and minimize the likelihood of bloating after eating.

Watch Out for Big, Fat, and "Tough" Meals

Big, fat, and tough may be great attributes for a bouncer, but they're the worst possible qualities in a meal when you're prone to sour stomach bloating. "Big" meals refer to large portions. Overeating is a surefire way to provoke an attack of sour stomach bloating. If you're prone to overdoing it at meals, it's important to eat regularly enough that you never arrive to the table feeling as though you're starving. If restaurant meals are your Achilles' heel, try asking for a take-out container to arrive along with your food so that you can pack up half the entrée before you start eating. Last, repeat after me: "Hara Hachi Bu." This is the Japanese diet trick of eating just until you are 80 percent full. This technique allows your brain to catch up with your belly so that you don't overeat before you've given your system enough time to register the feeling of fullness. It takes practice to master the art of stopping at 80 percent fullness, but keeping this goal at the forefront of your mind as you sit down to eat will likely slow you down and reduce the likelihood of overdoing it.

Fatty meals are a well-known cause of acid reflux, and they can trigger the sour stomach bloating that often accompanies it. Greasy take-out food, pizza with extra cheese, cheeseburgers with fries, pasta bathing in cream sauce, fried foods, and barbecue ribs are some of the high-fat staples of an American diet that are likely to provoke an attack of sour stomach bloating. I'm not suggesting that all high-fat foods need to be off limits if you're prone to sour stomach bloating, but what I do recommend is that you consume them as a "garnish" to an otherwise low-fat meal. Eating a slice of cheese on a turkey sandwich is quite different from eating an appetizer serving of deep-fried mozzarella sticks. Having a few slices of bacon on a BLT sandwich is quite different from having them on top of a greasy cheeseburger. Having a scoop or two of ice cream alone in a dish is different from having it atop a massive wedge of flourless chocolate cake. In other words, use higher-fat foods as garnishes to otherwise lower-fat meals rather than doubling up on them in a single sitting.

"Tough" meals refer to the texture of what you're eating. Think back to the metaphor I used in chapter 3, which portrayed your stomach as a blender. The stomach blender has to churn a whole lot longer to liquefy coarse-textured foods, such as salads, celery sticks, popcorn, and nuts than it does to liquefy soft-textured alternatives, such as cooked vegetables, soft corn tortillas, and peanut butter. Prolonged churning can increase the likelihood of reflux and the accompanying symptoms of upper-abdominal bloating. If you can't live without the crunch and would like to try to keep some tough-textured foods in your diet, here's how I recommend going about it:

- Avoid entrée-size salads or otherwise large portions of raw vegetables. Stick to side salads and appetizer-size portions.

- Eat your small appetizer-size salads at the end of the meal—just as the French do—rather than at the beginning of the meal, when your stomach contents are at their most acidic.

- Make salads from softer-textured "baby greens," such as spinach or butter lettuce, rather than tougher-textured leafy greens, such as kale, cabbage, frisée, romaine hearts, and iceberg lettuce.

- Pay attention to how you tolerate other coarse-textured foods, such as nuts and popcorn. Large portions are typically a recipe for trouble, though you may tolerate them in small portions, particularly when you've been eating in regular three-hour intervals. If even small portions bother you, then seek out the less-textured versions of these foods described in chapter 12.

- Chew all tough-textured foods exceedingly well. Pretend you're pre-chewing these foods for a toddler; each mouthful should be smooth and almost puréed before swallowing.

If the meal sizing and timing strategies described in this chapter don't alleviate your sour stomach bloating to a satisfactory degree, then I'd give the GI Gentle diet a try; it's described in chapter 12.

Don't Drink Alcohol on an Empty Stomach

Alcohol is a direct stomach irritant, and it also relaxes the gatekeeper muscle separating your stomach and esophagus. If you drink on an empty, relatively acidic stomach and you experience reflux afterward, it is going to feel mighty bad, and your sour stomach bloating may kick in after just a few sips. If you choose to drink alcohol, it's important to eat something small first. Eating decreases the acidity in your stomach and may help coat the mucous lining of your stomach as well. You'll also want to pace yourself while drinking and avoid drinking to excess. Last, if you're lying down in bed after a big, boozy night out, you'd be wise to leave some TUMS and an H2 blocker on your bedside table to pop in your mouth before you pass out. You'll thank me in the morning.

There's another type of belly bloat provoked by eating just like the sour stomach bloating described in this chapter, but unlike sour stomach bloating, it doesn't reliably respond to acid suppression. If this sounds familiar, read on to chapter 5 to see whether functional dyspepsia better describes your personal brand of bloating.

5.

The Distressed but Not Distended Bloat: Functional Dyspepsia

SOME TYPES OF BLOATING WITH roots in the stomach can feel a whole lot worse than they look from the outside. We spent chapter 3 discussing a few types of bloating that result in a visible increase in belly girth—a bulging appearance that almost makes sufferers look pregnant. But there's another type of bloating accompanied by a pressured, full feeling on the inside that does not correspond to much of a change in your belly's appearance on the outside. And unlike the sour stomach bloating described in chapter 4 that causes symptoms in the same upper part of the abdomen, this type of bloating is not associated with acid-related problems like reflux or heartburn. It's what experts refer to as *functional dyspepsia;* we'll call it FD for short.

Functional Dyspepsia (FD)

The term *functional* refers to the fact that FD is a condition caused by a stomach whose nerves and muscles don't operate as they should even though there's no structural disease affecting them. For example, you may feel gnawing discomfort in the upper part of your stomach, but your doctor can't find any evidence of ulcers, inflammation, or acid reflux that would cause this sensation. You might experience tightness, pressure, or the gurgling sound of gas moving around, but when your doctor examines you, there's no excess gas to be found. You might feel full after eating a small amount, but your stomach's emptying time turns out to be normal. Everything seems to be in order—so what could be causing this discomfort?

There are many explanations for the distinct upper-abdominal distress that people with FD experience. One likely cause of FD is the failure of your stomach to stretch properly after a meal. When empty, our stomachs are about the size of a closed fist. But when we start eating, they're supposed to be able to stretch significantly to fit a large volume of food. The stomachs of people with FD, however, may fail to relax sufficiently when food starts coming down the pipeline, and this failure to relax affects the upper region of the stomach in particular, making you feel uncomfortably overfull, even after a modest amount of food.

Another cause of bloating from FD may be disruptions in what's supposed to be a steady, evenly paced flow of food throughout the entire stomach. With FD, you may have normal stomach emptying time as measured by a gastric emptying scan (see chapter 3 for a description of this test), but the food you eat may linger a bit too long in the upper section of the stomach before moving on to the lower section. Alternatively, the impaired stomach stretch may actually cause the food you eat to rapidly dump into the lower portion of the stomach, since there's no room for it to linger up top. In this latter scenario, you might experience painful bloating in the lower region of the stomach.

Finally, people with FD may have an unusually high degree of sensitivity to things that stimulate the stomach, such as food, gas, or spices. While someone without FD wouldn't even feel a modest amount of gas passing through the upper stomach, someone with FD who has a heightened pain response in the digestive tract may experience the same amount of gas as incredibly uncomfortable.

What Bloating from Functional Dyspepsia Feels Like

Bloating from FD is usually concentrated in the upper part of the abdomen, right underneath the breastbone. My patients describe it as feeling uncomfortably full, tight, and pressured, and it's generally unchanged or worse after eating. The feeling of fullness doesn't always match the amount of food you've eaten; even a small amount of food can provoke feelings of being overfull. However, very large amounts of food or high-fat meals certainly make the symptoms much worse. The intensity of the bloating ranges widely; some people may only feel chronic, mild discomfort, while others complain of severe pain. Some people feel nauseated as well, but they don't generally vomit.

A big difference between FD and most of the other types of bloating that originate in the stomach is that it feels a lot worse than it looks on the outside. You may feel an unbelievable amount of fullness and pressure, but when your friend checks out your waistline, they'll insist you look like you normally do.

Another feature of bloating from FD is that it is *not* accompanied by heartburn, and it may only partly respond to medications that suppress acid, like Nexium, Prilosec, Zantac, and Pepcid—or not respond to them at all. While some patients may get minor but incomplete symptom relief when chewing calcium carbonate antacids, such as TUMS or Rolaids, it's usually because these meds happen to also trigger belching, which can relieve some painful pressure.

Last, bloating from FD is not accompanied by a change in bathroom habits, nor does it improve when you poop. Even people with FD who also happen to be chronically constipated won't feel much better in their upper-stomach regions if things improve for them in the bathroom. Bloating from FD is also not affected much by hormones; women seem to experience bloating at all times of their menstrual cycles without notable variation.

Diagnosing Functional Dyspepsia

Functional dyspepsia, like other functional disorders that affect the digestive system, is diagnosed based on a cluster of symptoms agreed upon by a committee of doctors from all over the globe. FD is what we call a *clinical diagnosis;* that means that there's no good test for it, and sometimes the diagnosis is made after other likely possibilities have been ruled out with available testing.

For example, if tests show that you have acid reflux, ulcers, or an infection from the bacteria called *H. pylori,* you wouldn't be diagnosed with FD, because there's an underlying disease that could account for your bloating. If tests show that you have delayed stomach emptying (or gastroparesis; see chapter 3), you wouldn't be diagnosed with FD, because your feelings of early fullness could be accounted for by an abnormally slow-to-empty stomach.

Assuming doctors have ruled out an underlying disease at the heart of your symptoms, they'll diagnose FD based on your report of chronic, persistent upper-abdominal discomfort that is unrelated to whatever is happening in the bathroom. But to get to this diagnosis, you'll likely have to undergo a few tests.

Endoscopy (EGD)

When you come in complaining of upper-abdominal pain and bloating, your doctor will probably want to check if this is an acid-related problem. Endoscopy is generally the first step in that process. As described in chapter 3, endoscopy is a procedure done under mild sedation. A gastroenterologist sends a tube with a camera attached through your mouth and down the esophagus, into your stomach, so he or she can see all of these organs from the inside. The test lasts only about fifteen minutes. By checking the appearance of your esophagus and stomach, and by taking some tissue samples in a procedure called a *biopsy,* your doctor can see whether there is inflammation or ulcers. Biopsies can also be analyzed for the presence of the irritating bacteria *H. pylori,* which causes inflammation and ulcers. If you have FD, the esophagus and stomach will look completely normal in this test.

Breath Testing for H. pylori

Sometimes instead of going straight to endoscopy, doctors will order a quick and noninvasive test of your breath to detect the presence of infection with *H. pylori*. If it's positive, they may treat you with antibiotics and see how your symptoms respond before considering the relatively more invasive (and definitely more expensive!) endoscopy.

You'll arrive after fasting at a gastroenterologist's office for your *H. pylori* breath test and swallow a pill or powder dissolved in liquid that contains a compound called *urea*. During the fifteen-minute test, you'll breathe into a tube so that the technician can capture and analyze samples of the gases in your breath. If you're infected with *H. pylori*, then your exhaled breath will contain all the clues needed to make the diagnosis. Blood testing for *H. pylori* is no longer recommended, because it can't distinguish between an active infection and a past infection that has since been resolved.

Esophageal pH Testing

Your doctor may want to verify if acid reflux accounts for your symptoms, and there are two tests he or she may use to do so. Both measure the pH level of your esophagus over a period of time.

The twenty-four-hour pH test involves monitoring the acid levels of your esophagus over a twenty-four-hour period and will often be the test of choice. It is done in your gastroenterologist's office, where he or she slides a thin tube up your nose and into your esophagus. At one tip of the tube is a little sensor that can measure pH levels in your esophagus. The other end of the tube, which is outside your body, is attached to a portable electronic recording device that you'll wear for twenty-four hours. The following day, you'll return to your doctor, the tube will be removed, and the doctor will take the recording device. The data contained within it will tell your doctor whether you've experienced acid reflux. If you have FD, then this test will come back normal and show no signs of acid reflux.

The Bravo test is another way doctors can detect acid reflux, and it provides the added benefit of checking the pH levels in your esophagus for a full forty-eight hours—twice as long as the twenty-four-hour test— to increase the chances of catching a correlation between your symptoms and pH levels in the esophagus. It is done during an endoscopy, while you're under sedation, and it involves your doctor attaching a small capsule to the lining of your esophagus. The capsule transmits data to a portable recording device that you'll keep on you for two days. You'll also keep a food diary during the test and record any symptoms you experience, such as heartburn. This test can be helpful in distinguishing whether your upper-abdominal pain or discomfort is related to reflux or functional dyspepsia, as your doctor can check the recording device to see if you were actually experiencing acid reflux at times you reported feeling upper-abdominal pain.

Gastric Emptying Scan

If your doctor suspects you may have delayed stomach emptying based on your description of feeling nauseated or full very quickly even after just eating a little bit of food, then he or she may order a test called a *gastric emptying scan* (GES), also known as *gastric emptying scintigraphy*. This test measures how long it takes food or liquid to pass through your stomach; it is described in full detail in chapter 3 in the section on gastroparesis.

People with FD will have a normal stomach emptying time, but sometimes a normal emptying test will pick up clues that point to FD by indicating how food flows through your stomach over time. For example, the radiologist administering the four-hour test might notice that it takes an abnormally long time for the food or liquid to progress from the top part of the stomach to the lower part of the stomach.

Treating Functional Dyspepsia

Medical Treatment for Functional Dyspepsia

A variety of both over-the-counter and prescription medications may help you manage bloating from FD, whether you take them on their own or in various combinations with one another. Based on the nature of your symptoms and your individual medical history, your doctor will recommend the most appropriate options for you to try. Generic medication names are provided in parentheses.

Over-the-Counter Medications

The least expensive, safest, and most accessible medications for relieving feelings of bloating, fullness, and tightness in the upper abdomen are surfactant drugs, such as Gas-X and Phazyme, or their generic store brands (simethicone). Surfactant medications work by breaking up large gas bubbles, which stretch the stomach, into smaller gas bubbles, which can move through the digestive tract more quickly. Some multitasking medications, such as Mylanta, combine simethicone with antacid ingredients; avoid mint-flavored varieties, as these can cause acid reflux.

Surfactant medications are not absorbed into the blood; they act locally in the digestive tract instead. This makes them very safe and easy to tolerate. In our practice, we advise patients with FD to try taking these medications *preventatively*, before starting to eat a meal, rather than waiting until they already feel bloated, after eating the meal. These medications can be taken several times per day before eating.

Serotonin-Blocking Medications

Certain medications bind to the receptors designated for a hormone called *serotonin* and mimic its calming and regulating effect on the nerves of the digestive system. They have been shown to be helpful in improving symptoms of FD. Specifically, they may improve stomach stretchiness after a meal and dull your hypersensitive abdominal pain response. These medications are developed and prescribed for a variety of other medical conditions but may have benefits when used off label (i.e., for unintended purposes), such as to manage the symptoms of FD.

One such medication is called *Zofran* (ondansetron), which is typically marketed as an antinausea and antivomiting drug. It's particularly helpful in managing chronic nausea among people with FD. It can be a bit constipating, but that's a side effect that can be dealt with. Another example is an antianxiety drug called *Buspar* (buspirone); it has a mild tranquilizing effect on the stomach muscles, relaxing the top part of the stomach and improving stomach stretch in response to meals. Typically, the medication is taken about fifteen minutes before eating a meal for maximum benefit. A popular migraine medication called *Imitrex* (sumatriptan) has also shown promise in relieving symptoms of FD. It may have more side effects than the alternatives, however, and it is not commonly used as a first-line treatment.

Antidepressants

Sometimes when doctors suggest antidepressant medications to address functional digestive system problems, my patients misinterpret this recommendation to mean that their doctor thinks they're crazy, or that the symptom is "all in their heads." This is not the case! Specific medications in a category called *tricyclic antidepressants* (TCAs) seem to have direct effects on the digestive tract by regulating levels of two hormones—serotonin and norepinephrine—that are involved in the pain response. Elavil (amitriptyline) is one of the more commonly prescribed medications used for this purpose, though its potential side effects, including constipation, make it difficult for some people to tolerate.

Prokinetic Medications

Prokinetic medications are designed to stimulate movement in the stomach, causing the stomach to contract more frequently so it will empty more rapidly and reduce feelings of bloating, fullness, poor appetite, and nausea. One such medication is Motilium (domperidone), which has shown the most promise in reducing symptoms. However, domperidone is not FDA approved for sale in the United States. Therefore, most American patients who use this drug import it from Canada or elsewhere overseas.

Dietary Treatment for Functional Dyspepsia

Dietary modifications alone are not a silver bullet for the bloating and discomfort from FD, but changing the way you eat can still make a major difference in the severity of your bloating and pain.

Eat Small, Soft-Textured, Low-Fat Meals

When you have FD, you should aim to choose foods and organize your meal patterns with a goal of limiting how much stretch you're causing your stomach at a given sitting. Smaller portions of food stretch the stomach less than larger portions; therefore, eating small amounts every three to four hours will provoke less bloating than eating three squares a day. Nighttime snacking after dinner is a common habit that can worsen bloating from FD. I've found that overeating at night often results from undereating in the earlier part of the day; my patients often fall into this pattern because they're afraid to provoke symptoms while they're at work, but it becomes a vicious cycle. This is why it's so important to figure out a tolerable grazing-type pattern during the day that enables you to feel more satisfied at night.

If you struggle to eat enough calories to keep you satisfied from these smaller meals, you can sip on nutritious liquids for hydration in between meals. Some examples include protein-fortified coconut waters or coffee drinks, water spiked with fruit-flavored protein powders, or a clear liquid meal replacement or protein drink (e.g., Ensure Clear, Boost Breeze, Isopure).

The texture of your food also plays a role in determining how much stretch you're asking of your rather rigid, extra-sensitive-to-stimuli stomach. Bulky foods rich in coarse-textured fiber can be very bloating and painful with FD; examples include salads (and raw vegetables in general), slaws, celery, popcorn, nuts and whole-nut snack bars, trail mixes, granola, and large portions of tough or leathery dried fruit. Bellies with FD prefer soft, smooth, creamy, mushy, and puréed textures. Your best-tolerated foods are likely going to be things like bananas, peanut butter, applesauce, papaya, yogurt, fruit smoothies, instant oatmeal, puréed vegetable soups, omelets, avocados, lean cold cuts like sliced deli turkey, and sushi. However, there is certainly room for some crunchy-textured foods in your diet, so long as they dissolve easily when chewed. Crunchy foods such as rice cakes, crackers, and many brands of breakfast cereals should go down pretty well.

Chapter 12 offers a detailed, extensive discussion of the soft-textured GI Gentle diet I recommend for FD, including lists of the friendliest and most problematic foods by food group. It also contains meal ideas and recipes. After finishing this chapter, flip ahead for more practical advice about which foods make great diet staples and which ones may give you trouble.

Sip Slowly and Don't Drink Liquids with Meals

Combining liquids with meals can result in excessive fullness in the upper part of the stomach. Some patients with FD also feel very nauseated when they drink liquids with a meal. In such cases, I recommend you stop drinking fifteen minutes before eating a meal and wait at least an hour after eating before drinking liquids for hydration.

You'll also want to make sure never to gulp, chug, or guzzle drinks. Instead, sip them slowly over the course of time, ideally using a straw. Dumping a large volume of liquid accompanied by extra swallowed air from gulping into your dyspeptic stomach is a surefire way to aggravate bloating. Sorry to be the bearer of bad news, but your days of chugging beer are over. Also, pay special attention to how you hydrate when exercising; it's common for people to gulp lots of water during a vigorous workout, and to swallow extra air when doing so, as the result of heavy, rapid breathing.

On the related topic of beverages, pay attention to how you feel after drinking coffee; it can aggravate the symptoms of some people with FD.

It may seem like a delicate balancing act to combine medications, meals, and liquids in a way that minimizes stimulating a stretch of the stomach. Trial and error will help you figure out a daily rhythm that best controls your symptoms, whether or not you have help from prescription medications. A sample daily rhythm may resemble something like the following:

SAMPLE WEEKDAY MEAL SCHEDULE FOR FUNCTIONAL DYSPEPSIA

SLOWLY DRINK YOUR MORNING COFFEE (IF TOLERABLE)/TEA/WATER: 6:30–7:30 A.M. after waking.

SIMETHICONE TABLET, THEN BREAKFAST: 7:45–8:30 A.M.

SIP WATER AS DESIRED FOR HYDRATION: 10:00–11:15 A.M.

SIMETHICONE TABLET, THEN SMALL LUNCH: 11:30 A.M. –12:30 P.M.

SIP WATER AS DESIRED FOR HYDRATION: 1:30–2:30 P.M.

MIDAFTERNOON SNACK: 2:45–3:30 P.M.

Avoid Stomach Irritants

Because some of the discomfort and pain from FD is caused by hypersensitive nerves, anything you put into your stomach that stimulates or irritates those nerve endings can worsen your symptoms. The most common stimulants include alcohol (all kinds) and spicy foods; these are best avoided as much as you are willing and able. Regular use of nonsteroidal anti-inflammatory drugs (NSAIDs), such as aspirin, ibuprofen, and naproxen, for pain relief can also be problematic, because they interfere with your stomach's ability to maintain its protective inner lining.

Anthony's Functional Dyspepsia Story:
A Lifetime of Feast-or-Famine Eating Finally Catches Up

Anthony was a gentleman in his late fifties who was referred to me by his gastroenterologist for symptoms of severe bloating after dinner almost every night. The problem had been going on for about ten months, though prior to this, he had a long history of acid reflux. Still, he insisted that this bloating problem was different from a reflux attack. Reflux attacks gave him heartburn, belching, and severe pain in the upper-right quadrant of his abdomen. This bloating problem was a different beast: no heartburn and no belching, but rather a feeling of fullness so uncomfortable that he'd find himself walking around the block for ages after dinner just to get relief. The bloating would kick in within minutes of eating, and it lasted for hours.

Anthony's doctor performed an endoscopy, and everything looked normal—there were no signs of acid reflux. Next, the doctor recommended Gas-X before dinner, but that didn't help. TUMS antacids didn't help either. After Anthony mentioned that he felt terrific after a recent business trip to Italy—where his eating schedule was very different from the one he follows at home—his doctor sent him my way to see if I could make sense of things.

When I met Anthony, he waxed nostalgic about his younger years. Throughout his thirties and forties, he'd hit the gym every morning, skip breakfast, skip lunch, and come home ravenous at around 5:30. He'd grab everything in sight to snack on until sitting down with his family to a home-cooked Italian meal later that evening—after which he'd feel full and satisfied, but not uncomfortable. But something changed in his fifties. That pattern of eating started putting weight on him—he'd gained thirty pounds over the course of the decade—and occasionally, he'd get attacks of heartburn and reflux-related pain from these nightly feasts. Red meat was especially problematic. In response to this change, he started grabbing a quick sandwich at lunchtime and eating a somewhat smaller, earlier dinner. This modified meal pattern seemed to help with the reflux.

But a few years later, despite no change in his diet, these new after-dinner bloating attacks started happening. As we walked through a typical day of Anthony's life, I learned that he'd start the day with a few coffees (and felt fine afterward) and then grab a tuna or roast beef sandwich around noon—plus a few cookies (and he still felt fine afterward). Dinner was usually eaten out at a restaurant, and by the time it rolled around at 7:00 P.M., Anthony would be starving. So he'd attack the bowl of bar nuts while he enjoyed a cocktail, and then he'd order a full entrée accompanied by two to three more glasses of wine. This meal pattern was starkly different from how he ate in Italy, where he'd start the day with a latte alongside a few rolls with butter and jam, followed about four hours later by a sit-down, two-course lunch of pasta and a fish-and-vegetable-based entrée. The portions, he noted, were more European in scale than American. At around 4:00 P.M., there was a coffee break, when Anthony would enjoy another latte with a few biscotti. By the time dinner rolled around at 8:00 P.M., he'd be only mildly hungry and eat a meal whose portion sizes were similar to those of lunch, alongside a single glass of wine.

Immediately, it was clear to me that Anthony felt best when he was eating more modest volumes of food every three to four hours or so, rather than allowing himself to be so hungry that he'd devour a huge amount of food in a single sitting at night. Less alcohol with dinner also seemed to sit better. For whatever reason, it seemed Anthony's stomach was extra sensitive to food and alcohol and no longer able to comfortably accommodate large volumes of food at once. As such, eating large volumes at night, coupled with four to five drinks, resulted in that feeling of excessive upper-abdominal fullness. Sounded like a likely case of functional dyspepsia.

I advised Anthony that it was time to start eating breakfast, lunch, and a midafternoon snack consistently so that his daily food intake would be evenly dispersed over the course of the day, rather than concentrated all at night. He needed to arrive at the dinner table a little hungry but not famished, so that he could control the amount he ate. I also suggested he stick to softer-textured foods, such as those on the GI Gentle diet (chapter 12) so that his stomach could empty a bit more expeditiously after eating and reduce the likelihood of a lingering overfull sensation. Finally, we took up Anthony's alcohol intake, and I suggested he'd be better off capping his nightly alcohol intake at two drinks, maximum.

I never saw Anthony again after this first meeting, so I assumed he didn't bother trying my recommendations—or perhaps that he had but hadn't found them helpful. It would be pretty hard to change a meal pattern that had been ingrained for so many decades, and it can be equally hard to cut back on alcohol, particularly in social settings. But three weeks later, I got a note from Anthony's gastroenterologist. Anthony had indeed implemented all of my recommendations and had reported feeling "worlds different—it was like night and day." His recurrent evening bloating and upper-abdominal discomfort were gone—and he had also lost five pounds to boot! The moral of the story is that extreme eating patterns eventually catch up to us all. Our digestive function often changes as we age, and sometimes we need to change the way we eat to accommodate it.

If your bloating experience definitely feels focused in the upper-abdominal neighborhood but is way belchier and less tied to eating than the conditions covered so far, then move on to the next chapter to see if aerophagia might be the problem.

6.

The Belchiest Bloat of All: Aerophagia

Aerophagia

Aerophagia is Latin for "swallowing air," and that pretty much sums up this entire condition. For one of a variety of reasons, you are prone to gulping down large pockets of air, which fill your stomach and cause uncomfortable pressure and distension. Whatever air you don't manage to belch out will continue traveling onward in your digestive tract, causing uncomfortable pressure and distension in the bowel until you are able to fart it out. This is because there's nitrogen gas in the air we breathe, which, if swallowed, cannot diffuse into the bloodstream and be exhaled through the lungs. If swallowed nitrogen gas is going to exit your body, it needs to be burped or farted out.

What Bloating from Aerophagia Feels Like

Aerophagia involves some degree of visible abdominal distension and is usually accompanied by a signature, telltale symptom: uncontrollable belching attacks. These are not demure, quiet little burps, mind you. They are loud, hearty, forceful belches that can strike seemingly out of the blue, and they often come in an uncontrollable, repetitive wave of a dozen or more belches per minute. In some cases, the belching can be constant, lasting all day long and interfering with work and social interactions. The bloating itself may be accompanied by sharp gas pains pretty much anywhere in the abdomen—upper or lower—depending on where in the digestive system your swallowed air is passing through.

People with aerophagia may be prone to swallowing air in their sleep, while talking, while eating or drinking, while singing opera, while smoking, or simply while walking around doing nothing but breathing. Because of this, bloating and belching from aerophagia can strike at any time of the day and may or may not be particularly associated with meals. It may be worse with stress. If your bloating *is* caused by swallowing air while you eat, then you may experience a belching attack within minutes of eating and possibly feel a bit short of breath as well. While aerophagia is commonly mistaken for acid reflux when it strikes after eating, it does not improve with any food eliminations or acid-reducing medications.

It is often the case that bloating from aerophagia is least noticeable in the morning and builds as the day progresses, but there are certainly exceptions in cases where the symptom is caused by swallowing air overnight while you sleep, like from snoring or use of a CPAP machine for sleep apnea.

Some people with aerophagia will also experience excessive farting, and it's not unheard of for them to become a bit constipated as the result of their bowel being distended from too much gas. Aerophagia is not triggered by certain types of food more so than others, unless you are prone to swallowing more air when you eat certain types of foods—like slurping down hot soup, for example.

Diagnosing Aerophagia

Your doctor may simply diagnose aerophagia based on interviewing you about your symptoms and when they strike, reviewing your medical history for risk factors, and/or witnessing a belching attack. He or she may order an x-ray of your abdomen, which will often show the presence of gas in the stomach or intestines. In some cases, your doctor may put you through an extensive battery of tests to rule out acid reflux or other diseases before landing on a diagnosis of aerophagia. In our practice, we may send a patient with suspected aerophagia to a specialist called a *speech language pathologist* (SLP) to have their swallowing function observed and evaluated for abnormalities that could account for an increased amount of swallowed air.

Treating Aerophagia

To treat aerophagia effectively, your doctor will need to figure out whether your problem is more behavioral or physiological and then tailor the treatment accordingly. If you have anxiety or obsessive-compulsive disorder (OCD), you may simply swallow saliva more frequently than normal, hyperventilate when feeling anxious, or develop other types of nervous tics—like sniffling—that can result in swallowing too much air. (This is surprisingly common in children who experience bloating, in fact.) If you're a runner or other endurance athlete, you may swallow air when exercising strenuously or when gulping down water at the gym. If you've got seasonal allergies or sinus issues that result in postnasal drip, you may be subconsciously sniffling all day long, swallowing air all the while.

On the physiological side of things, there may be something unusual about how you swallow that results in excessive swallowed air. If you use a CPAP machine for sleep apnea, the pressure settings might be inappropriate, resulting in forced air entering your esophagus (food pipe) instead of your air pipe; alternatively, you may be using the wrong type of mask.

Medical Treatment for Aerophagia

Medical treatments for aerophagia need to be tailored to the cause to be effective.

Behavioral Therapy

When the cause of aerophagia is behavioral, such as from hyperventilation triggered by anxiety, sometimes a type of therapy called *cognitive behavioral therapy* (CBT) is prescribed. Alternatively, learning techniques of diaphragmatic breathing—a slow, deep type of breathing—can also be helpful. You can learn diaphragmatic breathing in meditation classes or in consultation with a physical therapist, speech language pathologist, occupational therapist, or a cognitive behavioral therapist. There are loads of free instructional videos and illustrated step-by-step tutorials available online as well for you to view and practice.

Antianxiety Medications

In some cases, your doctor may recommend an antianxiety medication to help control some of the subconscious nervous tics that can cause aerophagia. There are many different options available, and the scientific research suggests that numerous options have been effective in patients with aerophagia. Your doctor will likely choose one based on your personal history and individual medical considerations.

Antispasmodic Medications

A few small studies have suggested that a muscle-relaxing medication called *baclofen* may be helpful in reducing bloating and belching among certain people with aerophagia whose symptoms are behavioral.

Surfactant Medications

As described in previous chapters, so-called surfactant drugs like Gas-X, Phazyme, and their generic store brands (simethicone) break up large gas bubbles in the digestive tract into smaller gas bubbles that can move through the digestive tract more quickly and cause less pain and distension on their way. I recommend that my patients take a simethicone tablet immediately *before* engaging in common trigger situations, like eating or exercising. These over-the-counter medications are safe to use several times per day.

Dietary (and Lifestyle) Treatment for Aerophagia

The following is a list of diet and lifestyle recommendations I make for my patients with aerophagia. These will only work for patients whose bloating is caused by swallowing air when eating, drinking, or smoking, however.

- Don't chew gum.

- Quit smoking.

- Drink liquids from a straw whenever possible.

- Eat slowly.

- Don't talk while chewing/eating.

- Tuck your chin down to your chest (as if you're looking down at your own belly button) when you are ready to swallow a mouthful of chewed food. This prevents air from being able to be swallowed along with the food.

Ellie's Aerophagia Story:
Attack of the Unrelenting Hiccups and Burps

Ellie was a twenty-eight-year-old woman who came to me by way of her gastroenterologist, to whom she turned with a curious problem: hiccups. Since starting a super-stressful job as a production assistant for a daily television show, she'd been plagued by relentless attacks of hiccups and loud belching. These attacks were accompanied by feelings of bloating and pressure-type pain in her upper abdomen—right underneath her breastbone. Sometimes she'd also hear sounds of gas swirling around in her lower belly, though her bowel movements were actually normal.

Ellie would wake up feeling fine and feel good after breakfast as well. Given how busy work was—there was barely time to take a bathroom break—she'd generally scarf down lunch at her desk within minutes. Immediately after, the bloating and belching attacks would come on, and they'd last for up to eight hours. She noticed that chewing any kind of gum would also bring on a terrible attack. Needless to say, these symptoms caused Ellie serious embarrassment at work. Over time, she learned that she could get the bloating to pass much more quickly if she drank a warm drink, lay down for a few minutes, and concentrated on deep, slow breathing, but this was not realistic at her fast-paced job, and it was getting to the point where she'd have to leave work early up to twice per week. Curiously, Ellie never had attacks on weekends, and she was racking her brain to figure out what she was doing differently to account for the change. Was it a difference in the food she ate on weekends? The amount of sleep she got? How quickly she ate her meals? Her stress levels?

Her doctor initially suspected the bloating, belching, and hiccuping were a result of acid reflux, possibly brought on by eating too much lunch too quickly or some component of her meals, like fat or garlic. But after trying out an acid-suppressing medication for a month and cutting out common acid reflux triggers from her diet—like garlic, onions, tomatoes, coffee, and chocolate—there was no change in her symptoms. So her doctor tried a different approach: a prescription antianxiety medication that also has an antispasm effect on the smooth muscles of the digestive tract. The medication definitely helped reduce the frequency and severity of her bloating and belching/hiccuping attacks, but it still wasn't a silver bullet.

Once Ellie told me her whole story, I was pretty suspicious that we were looking at a case of aerophagia. Because her symptoms appeared like clockwork after weekday lunch no matter what she ate—and never occurred on weekends no matter what she ate—it seemed unlikely to me that a particular food or ingredient was the culprit. Rather than being caused by *what* she ate, I suspected her bloating was being caused by *how* she ate. I believed she might be swallowing air when scarfing down her lunch in a frenzy—and possibly also due to a nervous swallowing tic as the result of feeling so stressed out at work all the time. The fact that Ellie had no symptoms on her (relaxed) weekends and that she could work through her symptoms when she paused for a few minutes to concentrate on deep, slow breathing were huge clues.

Based on these suspicions, we did a little experiment: For two weeks, Ellie agreed to chew a simethicone tablet (Gas-X) before eating anything, and she would tuck her chin down into her chest before swallowing food or drinks to prevent excess swallowed air.

For ten days, the simethicone and swallowing trick worked—and it worked well. She had 100 percent relief from symptoms for almost two glorious weeks. But then, her old bloating, belching, and hiccuping started resurfacing. Based on Ellie's promising response to the simethicone experiment, though, her doctor now knew exactly what to do: She prescribed a muscle-relaxant medication called *baclofen,* which is sometimes used to treat aerophagia, and sent Ellie to a cognitive behavioral therapist (CBT) to learn diaphragmatic breathing techniques. Adding the second medication did the trick; the bloating and belching attacks stopped completely and permanently. After Ellie has the opportunity to learn how to control her breathing and swallowing during stressful situations using CBT methods, though, her doctor is optimistic that she'll be able to wean Ellie off the medications that are giving her relief for now.

This chapter concludes the types of bloating that originate in the stomach. If nothing has struck a chord yet, fear not! We're headed toward the intestines, where there's plenty more bloating ground to cover!

PART III

LOWER-ABDOMINAL BLOATING THAT ORIGINATES IN THE INTESTINES

7.

The Backed-Up Bloat: Constipation-Related Bloating

IF YOU'VE MADE IT TO this section of the book, you're not convinced that your bloating has its roots in the stomach. So let's leap ahead to the tail end of the digestive process to see whether a colon full of stool may be the source of your bloating woes. As described in chapter 2, those of us in the digestive health world often refer to this as being FOS, which stands for "full of stool." (Or, depending on the bedside manner of your gastroenterologist, the *S* might stand for a more colorful alternative.)

The colon, also known as the large intestine, makes up the final segment of the gastrointestinal tract, and it's where waste is formed into stool and passed out of the body. To turn mushy leftover food waste into properly formed stools, the colon reabsorbs lots of extra water into the body. The longer your waste spends in the colon, the more water gets reabsorbed. This can cause stools to become *too* dried out and, therefore, quite hard to pass. The last several inches of your colon are a straight, muscular segment called the *rectum*. The rectum attaches to a round muscle called the *anus,* which should relax enough to allow you to defecate, but remain tight enough when you're not attempting to defecate so that any stool waiting on deck doesn't slip out by accident.

Constipation

Constipation can mean several different things, so it's important to be very specific when communicating about it to your doctor. It can refer to your experience when trying to move your bowels, like a chronic need to strain, or a feeling like you're not able to empty out completely when you do manage to go. It can also refer to the texture of your stool, like having chronically hard stools that may be long but lumpy, or passing hard, small little balls that look like rabbit pellets. It might also refer to the frequency with which you move your bowels: fewer than three times per week is considered constipation. Your symptoms may be a combination of some or all of these things. In other words, there are many different ways to be constipated, and even people who are able to poop something out on a daily basis can still be quite constipated.

Just as there are many different ways to be constipated, there are also many different causes of constipation. While all causes of constipation may produce similar symptoms, they will typically respond differently to various diets and medical treatments. For example, you may be constipated due to a basic lack of fiber in your diet, but your colon actually functions perfectly well. You may be constipated as a result of irritable bowel syndrome (IBS), which causes unpredictable patterns of movement in your colon. Perhaps your colon moves more slowly than normal, and that causes the stool passing through to become excessively dried out in transit. This is called *slow-transit constipation*. Using opioid pain medications can cause a type of slow-transit constipation called *opioid-induced constipation* (OIC).

Another under-recognized cause of constipation has to do with dysfunction of the nerves and muscles involved with defecation, causing what doctors refer to as an "outlet problem"; this is called *pelvic floor dysfunction* (PFD). One type of PFD, called *dyssynergia,* occurs when a slinglike muscle that supports your rectum contracts instead of relaxing when you try to poop. This pushes the stool backward rather than propelling it forward, leading to constipation and sometimes even blockages. Other types of PFD occur if the muscles involved in defecation are just too weak—say, from a childbirth injury—to push stool out efficiently. Alternatively, the anal muscle may be too tight to allow passage of stool easily and completely.

Whatever the nature of your PFD, it typically results in a form of constipation that doesn't respond particularly well to high-fiber diets or laxatives. You may have very infrequent bowel movements—like once per week, or even less often. Or you may go more frequently but have a very hard time pushing out your stool even when its texture is perfectly soft. You may constantly feel like your bowel movements are incomplete, as if there's more in there but you just can't get it out. People with certain types of PFD may have episodes of fecal incontinence, which means you are prone to having accidents where some amount of stool slips out without you realizing it. Other symptoms that may be associated with PFD are painful vaginal or anal intercourse; a very frequent, urgent need to urinate; chronic prostatitis (in men); and/or difficulty holding in urine. PFD is more common among people who also have a history of anxiety or emotional or sexual trauma; when this is the case, severe constipation may onset seemingly out of nowhere soon after an emotionally traumatic event. Women who have experienced prolonged labor or complicated vaginal deliveries of their children are also at higher risk of developing PFD. However, plenty of people with PFD have none of the above risk factors.

Finally, it's important to realize that even if you're able to have some sort of daily bowel movement, you can still become backed up with a colon full of stool. This happens if you create more daily stool volume from your high-fiber diet than you are able to eliminate through pooping. This is an under-recognized form of constipation, because the fact you're able to poop daily may lead you to believe that you couldn't possibly be constipated. However, the signs and symptoms of backed-up bloating described below should tip you off to the possibility.

What Bloating from Constipation Feels Like

Whatever the cause of your constipation, the bloating experience typically feels pretty similar. Backed-up bloating typically results in a distended belly that feels rock hard and that may deflate slightly after you poop, but rarely completely flattens. It is usually accompanied by attacks of lower-abdominal pain that kick in soon after eating a meal—especially large, high-fat, or high-fiber meals. This is often the result of trapped gas being propelled forward only to hit a bottleneck of poop that prevents you from farting it out. It may be spasmlike, crampy pain from a colon trying to advance the stool forward but unable to get it past the finish line and out of your body. There may also be pain after having a bowel movement, as if the colon or rectum is cramping up trying to eliminate more stool but is unable to do so.

People with backed-up bloating who are able to pass their gas often find themselves having farting attacks for hours each day, particularly almost immediately after eating larger meals like lunch and dinner, and the gas itself smells fecal (like poop) or sulfurous (like eggs). Constant, smelly gas is a common complaint among people with backed-up bloating.

The main way backed-up bloating is alleviated is if the "dam breaks" after a multiday stretch of not going to the bathroom. Let me explain: You may find yourself trapped in a cycle of multiday constipation where you struggle to poop at all, which culminates in a "washout" day where you find yourself running back and forth to the bathroom, having numerous, often crampy bowel movements in a row. The bowel movements may become increasingly softer, and even liquid, as the day progresses. At the end of this day, the bloating is fully relieved, and your belly feels notably flatter. However, as the constipation cycle restarts, the bloating starts building more and more by the day until it resumes its usual distended appearance. Sometimes the dam-breaking effect happens by itself; in other cases, you might bring it on by using laxatives to alleviate the worsening bloating sensation you experience with each passing day.

When backed-up bloating gets particularly bad, it may dampen your appetite or make you feel nauseated. Because you feel so full, the thought of putting food into your mouth may lose its appeal. Sometimes my patients describe feeling like the food in their stomachs has nowhere it can go, so it just "sits there." There is some truth to this perception; when the downstream segment of your digestive tract becomes clogged, it can certainly slow the flow of food and waste farther upstream in the digestive process.

Diagnosing Constipation

Bloating from constipation will only be alleviated once the constipation itself is alleviated. Constipation can generally be diagnosed based on a conversation with your doctor about your stool's appearance and how often you have a bowel movement. In addition, your doctor can often tell whether you're FOS by examining your bare belly by sight and by touch. To a trained eye, the outline of a colon full of poop is often visible from the outside, though if you're seeing a gastroenterologist, he or she is likely to conduct a rectal exam (this is described briefly farther along in this chapter). Most doctors will recommend diet changes, laxative regimens, and/or prescription medication based on a simple conversation and physical exam; they may also draw some blood to check your thyroid function, as an underactive thyroid (hypothyroidism) can produce slow-transit constipation as a side effect. If you respond well to these interventions, then it's unlikely your doctor will pursue any more invasive types of medical testing.

If your constipation does not respond satisfactorily to the first-line treatments—like a higher-fiber diet, over-the-counter laxatives, or even prescription medications—your doctor may pursue one or more tests to help understand the nature of your problem and its underlying cause so specific treatments can be tailored to you.

X-Ray

A simple x-ray of your abdomen, commonly referred to as a *KUB x-ray* (kidneys, ureters, and bladders x-ray), shows the burden of stool in your colon to reveal whether you are indeed FOS. This can be especially helpful when you show symptoms of constipation-related bloating but you're still able to have daily, regular bowel movements that might make you think you couldn't possibly be constipated. A doctor might also use such x-rays to identify whether you have something called *obstipation*, which is a blockage of the colon from a hard, dried-out bit of stool. People with obstipation may be chronically bloated and constipated but might suddenly begin to experience liquid diarrhea and possibly even fecal incontinence. This is called *overflow diarrhea*, and it results from the liquid waste from farther upstream in the bowel squeezing past the dried-out stool that's blocking your colon. Often, if you're obstipated and use laxatives to try to move your bowels, you can experience such overflow diarrhea, because the laxatives draw lots of fluid into the bowel, which builds pressure behind the blockage until some of the liquid forces its way out around the margins.

Motility Studies

Motility studies are multiday tests that your doctor uses to determine whether your bowel moves more slowly than normal. The normal time lapse from when you eat a food until the time you poop out what's left of it is anywhere from twenty to forty hours; your waste typically spends twelve to thirty-two of those hours in the colon itself. If matter takes longer than this to make its way through the colon, then your constipation may be related to slow transit.

A sitz marker study is a common motility test where you swallow a capsule containing tiny markers that your doctor can track via x-ray to see how long they take to move through your colon. A few days after swallowing the capsule, you return to the doctor for an x-ray of your abdomen to see whether any of the markers remain in your colon, and if so, how many. You may be asked to return again for another x-ray a few days later. This test can tell your doctor whether your colon is abnormally slow, and if so, to what extent.

Another test called *transenteric scintigraphy* allows your doctor to determine how long food spends traveling through each portion of your digestive tract: stomach, small intestine, and colon. It can be helpful if your doctor suspects there may be slowness affecting more than one segment of your digestive system. Based on where the delay(s) is/are, your doctor may be able to prescribe medications targeted to the problem area(s). As described in chapter 3, this multiday test requires you to be at the radiologist's office for six hours on the first day, where you will eat a bit of radiolabeled food, and then come back for a quick photograph every day for the next three days.

Defecography

Defecography is an imaging test using MRI technology that enables your doctor to see your pooping muscles in action. It is one way to diagnose problems with the various muscles of your so-called pelvic floor, which must coordinate in a specific way to enable you to pass stool effectively and completely. For women, a defecography can also identify whether there is a weakness in the muscular wall separating the rectum and vagina, called a *rectocele,* which causes the rectum to bulge into the vagina and form a "pocket" that might trap stool on its way out, preventing you from passing it completely. Defecography involves you lying in an MRI tube, where you will be asked to try pooping out a contrast substance that's been inserted into your rectum via enema prior to the test.

Manometry

Anorectal manometry is a short test that can be performed in a gastroenterologist's office, which measures the squeeze pressure, push pressure, and resting tension of your anus and rectum to see if they are interfering with your ability to poop normally. If these muscles are hypertensive (too tight), you might not be able to pass a stool normally. If they are hypotensive (too weak), you might not be able to propel a stool forward effectively, or you might be prone to incontinence of your gas or feces (pooping accidents). The test involves having a thin tube attached to a machine and covered in a balloon inserted into your rectum; the tube sends air into the balloon to inflate it. As you try to expel the balloon as if it were a poop, the machine's sensors can register your various muscles' pressure. The test is used to determine whether pelvic floor dysfunction is contributing to your constipation.

Rectal Exam

A gastroenterologist may conduct a rectal exam, in which he or she inserts a gloved, lubricated finger into your rectum and has you relax and squeeze your anal muscles, as well as bear down (push). The degree of squeeze and push pressures you are able to muster may offer a clue as to whether pelvic floor dysfunction is a likely possibility.

Treating Constipation

The most effective treatment for constipation will vary based on the specific cause. Typically, doctors will start conservatively by recommending a higher-fiber diet and/or some of the over-the-counter supplements or medications described below. Other remedies may be prescribed on an as-needed basis depending on your response and the results of any further testing.

Medical Treatments for IBS-Related Constipation or Slow-Transit Constipation

If you have chronic constipation for whatever reason, figuring out a regimen that helps keep you regular—and then sticking to it—is key to managing your backed-up bloating. Typically, the regimen will combine diet, supplements, and/or medications. Often, my patients will take liberties with their bowel regimen—sticking to it regularly when symptoms flare and then abandoning it when things are more regular. They do this out of fear of "becoming dependent" on supplements or medications. In my experience, however, consistency with the regimen—even when you're feeling good—is what *keeps* you feeling good. Besides, a great many modern laxative medications are not dependency-forming. In other words, most available options don't make your baseline bowel function any worse as the result of even long-term use.

Over-the-Counter Laxatives

There are many choices for over-the-counter laxatives, and they differ based on their mode of action. Osmotic laxatives work by attracting water into the colon (and keeping it there), which helps keep stool soft and speeds up its transit time toward the exit door. Laxatives in this category are not habit-forming, as they do not affect your colon's underlying function. Examples include MiraLAX (polyethylene glycol), magnesium (at doses of 350 milligrams or more), or Phillips' Milk of

Magnesia (a form of magnesium called *magnesium hydroxide*). Certain sugars that people cannot digest, such as lactulose and sorbitol, would also be included in this family, but because they can create so much gas, I tend not to recommend them to bloated patients unless they can't use most types of medicines for medical reasons, such as poor kidney or liver function. Osmotic laxatives take a good eight to twelve hours to kick in, so I recommend using them at night before bed to help you move your bowels the next morning. Very high-dose osmotic laxatives are also what doctors prescribe for the colon flush you're required to do before a colonoscopy. This should tip you off to the possibility that diarrhea is a possible side effect of osmotic laxatives if you overdo it, so you may need to experiment in order to find the perfect dose.

Stimulant laxatives work by affecting the function of the inner lining of the intestines, causing them to contract more regularly. As a result, some people find stimulant laxatives can produce more cramping than osmotic laxatives. Examples include Dulcolax (bisacodyl) and senna, which may be marketed in pills (e.g., Senokot) or in digestive teas sold under various names, such as Smooth Move. Stimulant laxatives work faster than osmotic laxatives, usually within a few hours. Still, you can take them before bed for results the following morning. It was once thought that stimulant laxatives were dependency-forming when used long term and could possibly affect your underlying bowel function in a way that would require increasing doses over time. However, there isn't much research to support this belief. Because osmotic laxatives are gentler and less likely to cause cramping, I steer my patients to them as a first-line treatment, but I suggest stimulant laxatives for occasional, temporary use to help them through a particularly rough patch when needed.

Fiber Supplements

Fiber helps people with sluggish colon motility or weaker pelvic floor muscles by bulking up their stools into plump, soft, and cohesive log-like poops. Soft, bulky stools stimulate the walls of the colon to keep pushing things along, and they are far easier to pass than hard little balls of dried-out poop. Commercially available fiber supplements use a variety of fibers known for their ability to absorb lots of water and plump up nicely in the gut. As this explanation suggests, it's important to take fiber supplements with plenty of water for them to work.

If you are very FOS, a fiber supplement is not the ideal first choice for your bowel regimen; it may worsen feelings of heaviness and bloating, until some of the backed-up stool is passed with the help of an osmotic laxative or other remedy. Some patients describe the experience of using a fiber supplement when they're already backed up with lots of stool as feeling like they've "swallowed a brick."

Supplements like psyllium husk—sold as a generic, but also under the Metamucil and Konsyl brand names—work well as bulking agents for constipated people, as does FiberCon (calcium polycarbophil). If you are prone to alternating bouts of diarrhea and constipation, products that are pure soluble fiber—such as Citrucel (methylcellulose), Benefiber (wheat dextrin), and acacia fiber—may be a better choice. These are all available in store-brand/generic and brand-name varieties. If you are taking a flavored fiber powder, note that some brands can have incredibly high amounts of sugar—up to four teaspoons per serving! In my experience, pills work just as well as powders, but pay attention to the dose size; you may need to take up to four pills to achieve a full two-gram dose of fiber, depending on the brand. See chapter 11 for a full discussion about the different properties of fiber, and chapter 14 for more details on specific types of fiber supplements.

I do not recommend fiber supplements routinely for people with constipation from pelvic floor dyssynergia, though certainly I have occasionally done so for individual patients on a case-by-case basis. When pelvic floor muscles aren't able to relax in order to pass stool effectively, piling on loads of fiber may just back you up even more. If you are someone who typically has only one bowel movement per week (or less), and for whom a variety of laxatives have not been effective in the past, a pelvic floor evaluation may be helpful. See the section below for constipation remedies specific to pelvic floor dysfunction.

Stool Softeners and Lubricants

One of the colon's main roles is to recycle fluid back into the body, and it does this by absorbing water from the digestive tract. Therefore, the longer your stool spends in the colon, the more dried out it's likely to become. Hard, dried-out stools can be harder to pass and in severe cases even cause a blockage. Some types of dietary fiber can hold on to moisture in a spongelike manner and keep your stools soft even under prolonged colonic travel times; see chapter 11 for the discussion on soluble fiber. But certain over-the-counter medications and supplements can help out as well.

Stool softeners such as Colace (docusate sodium) are a safe, gentle way to help your stools hold on to moisture, keeping them soft and easier to pass. Colace does not get absorbed into the body from the gut, so it is considered very safe for even pregnant and nursing women. Colace is not a laxative, however, in that it doesn't speed up the travel time of stool through the colon or make you go to the bathroom more frequently. It takes about twelve hours or more to start working, so many people use it regularly at night to help smooth things out in their morning routine.

Mineral oil is a slick, slippery substance that coats hard stools in your colon, lubricating them so they can slip out more easily. It is available over the counter, and it can be taken by mouth or included in an enema. Mineral oil is an effective short-term addition to a bowel regimen if your laxatives aren't working sufficiently or you've gotten plugged up by a dried-out bit of stool—like, say, after returning from a vacation when your bowel habits were thrown way off. However, taking mineral oil by mouth is not a good choice for regular, long-term use. This is because it can interfere with your body's ability to absorb certain vitamins as it passes through the small intestine. I typically recommend my patients use it once per day for no more than a week straight to help make it through a rough patch.

Enemas

In rare cases, people can experience an extreme form of slow colon motility called *colonic inertia*. If you have colonic inertia, you may not respond adequately to any of the typical laxatives or prescription medications, even when they're combined and taken at high doses. In such cases, using over-the-counter enemas may be your best bet for relief from bloating. Enemas involve squirting a liquid preparation directly into your colon via the rectum to help loosen stool in the colon and flush some of it out. Often the enema liquid will contain some dissolved substances that have laxative properties and boost the treatment's effectiveness. One of the most common brands in the United States is Fleet, which markets several types of enemas, including osmotic (saline), stimulant (biscodyl), and lubricating (mineral oil). Generic and store-brand alternatives are widely available. People with colonic inertia or pelvic floor dyssynergia (see below) often find that using enemas regularly is the best way to get relief from constipation and bloating, because they deliver the effective ingredients directly to the last segment of the colon without having to traverse a prolonged journey through the slow and dysfunctional bowel. Enemas typically start working within minutes.

I do not recommend colonics done at spas, or even by dedicated colonic practitioners, in place of enemas. A colonic treatment, which is often marketed as "colon hydrotherapy," is a turbocharged enema that uses a machine to force water far deeper into your colon than a home-administered enema can reach. Most states do not license practitioners of colonics, which calls into question whether the person administering this procedure is well trained, capable, or qualified to do so safely. The combination of inserting machinery into the delicate tissue of your rectum and the forcefulness of the flow of water into your colon involves risk of tearing (perforation), and such perforations can be life threatening. Even when administered safely, regular colonics will disrupt the normal balance of bacteria that live in your colon and can actually worsen your baseline digestive function (and overall health) as a result. Finally, on the topic of bacteria, colonics equipment may not be cleaned and sterilized in the same regulated manner as the scopes employed by physicians administering colonoscopies. As one of my gastroenterologist colleagues quips, having a colonic can be like getting a free fecal transplant from an unknown donor. Buyer, beware.

Prescription Medications

When diet changes and over-the-counter medications aren't making a dent in your chronic constipation, your doctor might suggest trying one of a few prescription medications. Amitiza (lubiprostone) is one such drug, which works by changing the secretions of the cells lining your colon in a manner that softens stools and increases spontaneous movement of the bowel. It is not dependency-forming, and when you stop using it, your colon will revert to its baseline level of activity. Another option is called *Linzess* (linaclotide), which also acts on the cells lining the colon, increasing secretions of fluid that soften stool and stimulating the nerves that promote contractions of the bowel that move stool along. Its most common side effect is diarrhea. The most recent constipation medication to be approved by the FDA is called *Trulance* (plecanatide). It works in a manner similar to Linzess, by increasing secretions by the cells lining your colon, which have the effect of stimulating motility and softening stools.

Surgery for Constipation

In extreme cases of constipation—where no combination of diet change, medications, or enemas can provide adequate relief from symptoms that are severe enough to make a significant dent in your quality of life—your doctor might suggest surgery to remove part of your entire colon. This surgery is called a *partial* or *total colectomy*. In some cases, the remaining part of the bowel is reattached to the rectum and keeps the general plumbing intact. In other cases, the remaining bowel is routed outside the body through an ostomy. If you have an ostomy, then immediately following the surgery, waste will empty into a bag you wear outside your body called an *ostomy bag*. After the surgical site heals, a second surgery can often be performed in which the small intestine or remaining segment of colon is connected to the rectum, forming a small reservoir pouch to help hold stool. This allows you to go to the bathroom in the normal anatomical manner, commonly four to six times per day once healing is complete. If you are considering surgery, I urge you to consult with a colorectal surgeon who is well versed in motility disorders.

Medical Treatment for Constipation from
Pelvic Floor Dysfunction (PFD)

If the muscles involved with defecation aren't able to help you pass stool effectively, then loading up on fiber and laxatives may just stress a broken system and worsen your bloating. If your doctor suspects or has confirmed you have PFD, he or she may recommend some of the following treatments instead:

Keep a Step Stool in the Bathroom for Squatting

Changing your position when you sit on the toilet so that your body is in more of a squatting position while pooping can be helpful to all of us, but especially so when you have PFD. Squatting reduces the need for straining to pass your stool, and may be especially helpful when weaker muscle tone is the underlying issue. Placing a step stool in front of your toilet to rest your feet on will naturally elevate your knees and position your body from a more sitting-upright position to a more squatting-type position. While some entrepreneurial types market a specialized product for this purpose—the so-called Squatty Potty—I've found that any old step stool works for my patients just fine.

Rectal Glycerin Suppositories

Rectal suppositories are little bullet-shaped, waxy doses of medicine that you insert into the tail end of your colon through your rectum. Glycerin suppositories in particular attract water into this segment of the colon through osmosis and stimulate movement to help you pass some stool. They can be an effective way to get the benefits of an osmotic laxative if your colon motility is very slow or the muscles associated with defecation are not functioning properly. They are less messy to use than a liquid enema and usually produce results within an hour of inserting. However, they can be irritating to the skin of your anus if you use them regularly for more than a week straight. The Fleet brand markets glycerin suppositories, but they are widely available as generic brands as well.

Enemas

Enemas can be a helpful way to alleviate backed-up bloating while you're in the process of pursuing a more permanent solution, like physical therapy, biofeedback, or Botox, described below. See the previous subsection on enemas (page 89) for more details.

Pelvic Floor Physical Therapy/Biofeedback

If you've been diagnosed with PFD, a type of therapy called *biofeedback* can be helpful when combined with physical therapy to retrain the nerves and muscles associated with defecation to function properly. This therapy, which is also described in chapter 3, involves a trained therapist attaching sensors to your anal muscles as he or she guides you through a series of exercises designed to get you relaxing and contracting them. When the muscles coordinate properly, the sensors will produce either a graphic display on a video monitor or an audio cue that gives you feedback (hence the name) that you've gotten it right. Then you can practice that movement until you begin to have more control over it.

Botulinum Toxin (Botox)

If your constipation is being caused by anal muscles that are too tight and can't relax properly, one treatment option is to undergo Botox injections. The injections are typically done by a colorectal surgeon when you're sedated, and their effects should last several months.

Dietary Treatments for Constipation

For all types of constipation—with the notable exception of PFD—dietary changes can be very helpful in alleviating constipation and backed-up bloating.

Eat Larger, Consolidated Meals Rather Than Small, Frequent Meals

One way to stimulate your colon to get it moving is by triggering a nerve signal called the *gastrocolic reflex* (GCR). The GCR is a digestive messaging system in which the upstream stomach warns the downstream colon that a big meal is coming down the pipeline. This causes the colon to start clearing out space for the incoming food by moving waste (stool) onward and outward. Stretch receptors located on the stomach wall detect how full the stomach is getting from a meal and trigger the GCR in response to this physical stretch. Greater stretch triggers a stronger response. This explains why many people often feel the need to have a bowel movement within an hour of eating a particularly large meal.

If you want to take advantage of this natural digestive system signaling tool, then you're best off eating three more sizable meals per day instead of grazing on small meals and snacks every few hours. Larger meals activate that stomach stretch and get the colon moving; mini meals are less likely to do so. Similarly, eating bulky, voluminous foods like salads, popcorn, and even large portions of soup can do the trick.

Sample High-Fiber Diet Day for Women

BREAKFAST: 12 GRAMS FIBER

Oatmeal made from ½ cup dry rolled oats, cooked in water

2 tablespoons ground flaxseeds sprinkled into oatmeal

1 cup blueberries

Coffee! (Decaf works too)

LUNCH: 7 GRAMS FIBER

Open-faced turkey avocado sandwich on 1 slice whole-wheat bread

Small salad with greens and mixed vegetables (about 3 cups); dressing of your choice

DINNER: 7 GRAMS FIBER

Baked or broiled salmon

1 medium sweet potato

1.5 cups cooked green beans

SNACKS: 7 GRAMS FIBER

2 kiwis

¼ cup nuts

Gradually Ramp Up Your Fiber Intake

The definition of *fiber* is a carbohydrate from plant-based foods that humans lack the digestive enzymes to break down. Because we can't break fiber down to release its stored energy (calories), it stays in the intestines and travels on to the colon where it will eventually be pooped out. If you're not eating enough fiber, then you'll struggle to have enough substance in your colon to produce regular, complete, easy-to-pass bowel movements. Or as I remind my patients: nothing in, nothing out.

Patients often ask me, "How much fiber should I be eating?" It's a tricky question to answer, as there's no single magic number that works for everyone. Some people may require significantly more dietary fiber than others to stay regular in the bathroom, so the trick is to start gradually increasing your intake until you notice things changing for the better. Keeping an electronic food journal can be really helpful in identifying your personal magic number to target, as most available apps automatically tally your fiber intake when you record your food. A good place to start would be to aim for *at least* 28 grams per day for women and 38 grams per day for men.

Sample High-Fiber Diet Day for Men

BREAKFAST: 12 GRAMS FIBER

Mixed-vegetable omelet topped with ½ avocado, sliced

Two slices whole-wheat toast

Cup of pineapple chunks

Coffee!

LUNCH: 8 GRAMS FIBER

Asian-style salad from fast-casual restaurant chain (e.g., Chinese chicken salad or Thai salad with peanut vinaigrette)

DINNER: 14 GRAMS FIBER

Stir-fried mixed vegetables (2 cups cooked, frozen OK)

1 cup brown rice

¼ cup cashews or peanuts

Protein of your choice (e.g., chicken, steak, shrimp)

SNACKS: 9 GRAMS FIBER

100-calorie bag of popcorn

Large pear

When you're ramping up your fiber intake, you'll be much more comfortable doing so gradually. This is because a very high-fiber meal may make your bloating worse (and set off a gas attack) if you're particularly backed up. I suggest starting by increasing fiber intake at breakfast first. Morning is the time of day when you're likely to be the least bloated, and it's also when people are most likely to move their bowels, which provides some relief. (This is particularly so if you've taken a laxative the previous night and are sipping on a cup of coffee!) Once you've acclimated to a high-fiber breakfast, you can move on to boosting the fiber content of other meals and snacks, one at a time.

Another thing to consider when transitioning to a higher-fiber diet when you're still backed up with lots of stool is to skew your fiber-rich food choices to those relatively less likely to cause gas. Such foods are called *lower FODMAP*, and examples of them are described in great detail in both chapters 11 and 13. Once you are able to start emptying your bowels more regularly and completely, those favorite foods known to be on the gassier side—such as cauliflower, beans, or dried fruit— may be far less bothersome to you.

Watch Out for Processed Foods with Added Fiber, Particularly Inulin

When trying to increase your fiber intake, it can be tempting to try a processed food fortified with loads of added fiber—like high-fiber cereals and bars—that meet half of your daily fiber quota in just one sitting. So efficient, right? If you've got backed-up bloating, though, these fortified-fiber foods may make you feel pretty awful. That's because the most common source of fiber they contain is inulin, which may also be listed as chicory root fiber, Jerusalem artichoke fiber, or yacon syrup. No matter what name it goes by, inulin is highly fermentable by the resident bacteria in your colon, which means they produce a whole lot of gas when they encounter it. If you're truly FOS, then all that gas is likely to get trapped and make your bloating and gas pain worse, not better. Inulin is also a common additive to low-carb pastas, low-calorie yogurts, low-calorie frozen treats, granola bars, whole-nut bars, some probiotic supplements, and protein powders, so it's worth reading the labels of packaged foods you buy regularly.

Drink Coffee (Even Decaf)

If you're very constipated and you don't drink coffee, you might consider starting to do so. Coffee contains a substance called *chlorogenic acid*, which stimulates motility in the colon. Your bowel is primed to poop each morning before 10:00 A.M. as the result of natural peaks in the stress hormone cortisol, whose job it is to wake your sleepy bowel and transition it to active daytime mode. A well-timed dose of chlorogenic acid, delivered via your morning coffee, may pile on an extra bit of oomph to the effects of cortisol and get that bowel moving.

If you avoid coffee due to the side effects of caffeine, you can still get (some of) the benefits of chlorogenic acid even by drinking decaf. If you avoid coffee because it gives you acid reflux, see if you can tolerate it better about an hour after eating breakfast rather than immediately upon waking up. You can also try consuming coffee in latte form; the large volume of milk relative to coffee will buffer the acidity of your cup of joe, and for some people, this is enough to make it tolerable. If you're lactose intolerant, use lactose-free milk, coconut milk, or almond milk in your latte. I'd skip the soy milk; it's basically bean juice and can be quite gassy in its own right.

Try Supplementing Magnesium

Many of my constipated patients prefer to avoid medications but are open to supplementing a nutrient they happen to need anyway: magnesium. Magnesium is an essential mineral and electrolyte with benefits for heart health, bone health, and even headache prevention. When you supplement magnesium at doses of 350 milligrams or more, however, it has a laxative effect by drawing fluid into the bowel. For many of my constipated patients whose kidneys work well, taking 400–800 milligrams of magnesium in the evening is the little extra push they need to get things moving in the bathroom the following morning. (If you are elderly or your kidney function is compromised, then magnesium may not be an appropriate supplement for you, so please check with your doctor.) To try out magnesium, start with a 400-milligram dose for three evenings in a row. If it's not doing the trick, add an additional 200 milligrams per night and wait another three days. If you get to 800 milligrams and there's still no effect on your bowels, then you may need to switch tactics. Do not divide the doses into two separate sittings or you'll dilute the impact. The main side effect of too much magnesium is diarrhea; if you experience this, then just skip a day and try again at a lower dose the following evening.

Diana's Constipation Story: The Magic of Fiber and Magnesium

Diana was a fifty-two-year-old executive who consulted me as a "last resort" for her bloating. It had been going on for four years, she felt that she had tried everything, and she was very skeptical that anything dietary was going to help. But since her gastroenterologist had insisted, she begrudgingly agreed to give me a chance.

Diana's bloating saga started several years earlier, after a sudden attack of diverticulitis—an inflammation of some small, bulging herniations in her colon wall—that landed her in the hospital. Once she recovered, she noticed that she'd become quite bloated and constipated. Diana complained that she could only have a bowel movement once every three to four days—and on the rare occasions she went more frequently, she only managed to pass very small little balls of stool that provided minimal relief. Her doctor at the time told her she needed to consume 25 grams of fiber per day, and Diana tried to follow this advice by consuming prune juice, high-fiber cereals, and split-pea soups. But this diet left her unbearably gassy, with worse bloating than ever, and she couldn't stick with it. Her next doctor tried her on a variety of over-the-counter laxatives—including MiraLAX and magnesium—and then escalated her to prescription drugs for constipation. Diana felt that these drugs didn't work reliably to alleviate her constipation—and, by association, her bloating—so she stopped those too.

I understood why Diana felt she had tried everything to no avail, but after taking a diet history, I didn't agree. A typical day in Diana's life started with a yogurt or grapefruit juice for breakfast, paired with a latte (fiber count = 0 grams). Lunchtime was either a tuna sandwich on rye (fiber count = 3 grams) or a chicken noodle soup with oyster crackers (fiber count = 0 grams). Dinner was a nice balanced meal that started with a salad and was followed by an entrée of protein, starch, and some cooked veggies. But although this dinner contained a respectable amount of fiber-rich veggies, it was too little too late. While Diana had attempted a high-fiber diet before, she had chosen the absolute highest-FODMAP sources of fiber (see chapter 11)— it's no wonder she found it so unbearably gassy and bloat-inducing! And while she had attempted laxative medications of all varieties, she hadn't ever done so while also consuming an adequate amount of fiber.

Alleviating Diana's backed-up bloating was going to require getting her to poop a satisfying amount every single day. And since morning is often prime pooping time for many people, I felt she'd probably benefit from starting off the day with a substantial, fiber-rich breakfast to stimulate her gastrocolic reflex (see page 93). This morning meal should be followed by a fiber-containing lunch, and then her usual dinner. In the beginning, I told Diana that all of her fiber choices should be from lower-FODMAP fruits, veggies, and whole grains so that she wouldn't run into the same gassy bloat she'd experienced in her last go-around with a high-fiber diet. Once she was moving her bowels consistently, though, and there was less risk of having gas trapped behind a colon full of stool, I suspected she'd tolerate even higher-FODMAP foods. Last, I recommended Diana resume her old magnesium regimen each night before bed.

I could tell Diana was not optimistic about our plan, as she felt she had done all of this before. But she hadn't done it all at once in a layered approach, and she hadn't done it with consideration for FODMAPs. I implored her to follow my plan faithfully for two weeks before dismissing it, and she agreed. We came up with some meal ideas together: Breakfast would now be scrambled eggs with a big bowl of low-FODMAP fruit—melon, pineapple, and berries—along with a slice of whole-wheat sourdough toast. At lunch, she'd pair her usual sandwich with a side of baby carrots or grape tomatoes. No change to her usual dinner. If she wanted her favorite yogurt for a snack, she'd throw in some ground flaxseeds and berries. Finally, she agreed to be consistent with bedtime magnesium supplements.

Within three days, Diana was having complete bowel movements just minutes after finishing her big, fuller breakfast with coffee. The extra stimulus that her nightly magnesium regimen piled on to a diet that was now adequate in fiber and a morning meal that was big enough to spur her colon into action turned out to be the winning formula. And just as predicted, once she was pooping every day, the bloating was gone. Diana called me two weeks later to share the good news and asked how to proceed. I told her she needed to habituate the nightly magnesium, big breakfast, and inclusion of fiber-rich foods at each meal. But going forward, she should feel free to experiment with including some favorite high-FODMAP foods, such as bean soups, cauliflower, and cashews. It was very likely that she'd tolerate these foods comfortably now that her backed-up bloating was a thing of the past.

Diana's case illustrates the importance of a multipronged strategy to address constipation-related bloating. It often requires some balance of diet and laxative supplements or medication to alleviate the problem. It also speaks to the importance of choosing your fiber thoughtfully, as some types can actually worsen symptoms of bloating when your colon is backed up and full of stool. See chapter 11 for a more detailed discussion of this.

If you haven't yet recognized your brand of bloating, don't fret. We're now heading back upstream to the small intestine to describe the type of bloating that ensues when too many of your colon's resident bacteria set up shop in the wrong neighborhood.

8.

The Bacterial Bloat: Small Intestinal Bacterial Overgrowth (SIBO)

THE EPICENTER OF GAS PRODUCTION in our bodies is the large intestine, otherwise known as the colon, which was our focus in the previous chapter. This is because the colon is home to the largest and most concentrated population of bacteria in our bodies. These bacteria are the ones that produce most of the gas we end up farting out. The colon is next-door neighbors with the small intestine, the part of the gastrointestinal tract that connects the stomach to the colon. The small intestine is where most of the nutrients from our food are absorbed, and there aren't supposed to be too many bacteria living there. Under certain circumstances, however, the small intestine may become hospitable to bacteria, and they can develop excessively large populations. This condition is called *small intestinal bacterial overgrowth*, which we will call *SIBO* for short.

SIBO

The best way I can describe SIBO is "too many bacteria living in the wrong neighborhood of your gut." Contrary to common internet-fueled myths, SIBO is *not* a case of having "bad," disease-causing bacteria living in the small intestine. In fact, SIBO is not even considered an infection, nor is it inflammatory. Rather, SIBO is a situation in which the normal, usually harmless bacteria that typically reside in your colon somehow gain a foothold in the small intestine, where they don't belong in any great number.

This is a very important distinction, because the internet is brimming with sites marketing probiotic and other dietary supplement regimens promising to correct the balance of "bad bacteria" to "good bacteria" that they claim cause SIBO, or to "heal the gut" from what is characterized as inflammation-induced leakiness from SIBO. These are profound mischaracterizations of SIBO. In fact, if your small intestine is prone to overgrowing bacteria for whatever reason, it is possible (and even likely) that taking probiotic supplements full of bacteria could make the problem *worse*, not better.

So what might cause bacteria to overgrow in the wrong neighborhood of the gut? Researchers have identified dozens of possible risk factors. Some of the more common ones include the following:

- Chronic use of a "PPI" acid-suppressing medication, like Nexium, Prilosec, Prevacid, Protonix, Aciphex, Dexilant, or any generic version that has the suffix *-prazole*

- Having low levels of stomach acid, either from old age or because of an autoimmune disease like atrophic gastritis or pernicious anemia

- Abnormally slow motility (patterns of movement) in your small intestine

- Taking probiotic supplements when you also have one of the risk factors listed above

- Prior intestinal surgeries, such as Roux-en-Y gastric bypass for weight loss, a resection of your bowel at the border of the small intestine and colon, or any abdominal surgery that resulted in scar-tissue adhesions that affect motility in your bowel

- Inflammation in the section of your bowel at the border of the small intestine and colon (called *ileitis*), such as from Crohn's disease

- Undiagnosed or poorly controlled celiac disease

- Insufficient production of digestive enzymes by your pancreas (pancreatic insufficiency)

- Regular, heavy alcohol consumption

- A little outpouching in your small intestine called a *diverticulum,* in which bacteria can hide

- Extensive prior antibiotic exposure

As the list above suggests, SIBO is a symptom of another health issue rather than something that just occurs spontaneously. If you happen to be diagnosed with it, you'll need to talk to your doctor about identifying the underlying cause so that you can prevent it from happening again!

Whatever the reason you developed SIBO, the way it affects you is likely the same. After eating, your small intestine is full of food whose nutrients are in the process of being absorbed into the bloodstream. As large populations of bacteria come into contact with these nutrients, they start feasting. When bacteria digest food—and carbohydrates are the food group they like best—it is called *fermentation.* One end product of fermentation is gas, and it's this gas that contributes to the miserable bloating experience associated with SIBO. Furthermore, because the small intestine is so much narrower than the colon, it's far more uncomfortable when it fills up with gas. In more severe cases, SIBO also interferes with the body's bile-recycling system and permits excess bile—a fluid that helps with fat digestion—to accumulate in the colon. This is called *bile acid malabsorption,* and it can result in both diarrhea and certain vitamin deficiencies.

What Bloating from SIBO Feels Like

Bloating from SIBO often seems to appear one day as if out of nowhere. While you may have experienced mild bloating here and there, you've never felt this severely bloated this consistently. Foods and meals that once felt fine suddenly trigger significant reactions within an hour of eating them. The foods most likely to trigger a response are high-fat meals, like fried foods, creamy or cheesy dishes, ice cream, or greasier take-out meals. Wheat-based foods—such as bread or sandwiches, baked treats, pasta, and pizza—are also common triggers, as are almost all energy bars and granola bars. Chickpeas, beans, and typically "gassy" vegetables such as broccoli, brussels sprouts, and cauliflower are problematic too. For some people, certain fruits and dairy foods will suddenly bother them as well. Given how extensive this list is, you can understand why I commonly hear "Everything bloats me" from my patients with SIBO.

Most people with SIBO complain of having lots of intestinal gas, which can be quite painful. Sometimes the gas produces a distended-looking belly, and sometimes it just results in lots of farting, sharp pain, and/or the gurgling sound and sensation of gas moving around the gut somewhere beneath the belly button. Farts are often very foul smelling; some patients describe them as "toxic." Typically, mornings are the best time of day, with minimal to no bloating upon waking up, but as the day progresses and you eat more and more meals, the gas and bloating continue to build. After dinner is typically the peak bloating time; my patients are often unbuttoning their pants and farting up a storm until bedtime. With SIBO, the less you eat, the better you feel.

In most cases—but not all—SIBO is also accompanied by a change in your bathroom habits. The nature of the change typically depends on what type of bacteria you're overgrowing. People who harbor hydrogen-gas-producing bacteria are more likely to experience diarrhea and/or softer, more frequent bowel movements. Some of my patients find they have the urge to poop immediately after eating anything. There may also be a change in the color and texture of your stool; it can be lighter brown or more orange than usual, and often, it takes on a sticky, "toothpaste" or "tarlike" texture that is very hard to pass completely and difficult to wipe clean from your bottom. Some people describe their stools as feeling "acidic," like they irritate the skin on the way out, and often, they can leave a feeling of anal itching behind.

It is also possible for SIBO to cause constipation rather than diarrhea, and this is more common among people who are overgrowing

organisms that produce methane gas. My patients who become constipated with SIBO often find their bloating to be especially painful, because
the extra gas feels like it's trapped behind backed-up stool and can't be
alleviated by farting. The constipation typically responds well to mild
laxatives and/or a low-FODMAP diet; see below for more information.

While SIBO typically announces itself in terms of *lower*-digestive-
system complaints, such as farting and irregular bathroom patterns,
some people experience more symptoms in their *upper*-digestive systems
as well. For example, acid reflux, nausea, belching, or loss of appetite can
also accompany SIBO in addition to or instead of the lower-digestive-
system symptoms. Some symptoms of SIBO may have nothing to do
with the digestive system at all; unexplained vitamin B_{12} deficiency is a
common side effect of SIBO. Less common—but not unheard of—is for
people to experience something called *rebound hypoglycemia*, where their
blood sugar levels crash soon after eating refined carbohydrates or foods
high in sugar, leaving them feeling exhausted, dizzy, or nauseated.

Diagnosing SIBO

If you've experienced the type of bloating or any of the accompanying symptoms described above, your doctor may consider testing you for
SIBO. Often, he or she will also be looking for other possible explanations for your symptoms, such as celiac disease (blood test), low pancreatic enzyme levels (stool test), infection with a parasite called *giardia*
(blood and/or stool test), and inflammatory bowel diseases such as Crohn's
or colitis (colonoscopy). It's important to note that these medical issues
are not either-or: you can have Crohn's disease, celiac disease, or pancreatic insufficiency *in addition to* SIBO, especially because the former
may be the cause of the latter.

Breath Tests

The most common, least invasive way to diagnose SIBO is through
breath testing. The test requires you to drink a sugar solution, breathe
into a bag periodically over three hours, and have your breath gases measured by a machine. A proper test should measure two types of gases:
hydrogen and methane. Since only bacterial cells will produce these gases

when they encounter the sugar you drank, if the gases are on your breath, we know that bacteria made them. Based on the point during the test at which the gases show up, your doctor can determine where those bacteria are hanging out in your digestive system. And based on the types of gas that show up on your breath, your doctor can tell which type of critters you're overgrowing.

The accuracy of your breath test in diagnosing SIBO will depend on many factors, so it's important to follow the prep instructions you're given by the testing facility. For example, if you've taken antibiotics or had a "colon purge," such as colonics or colonoscopy within four weeks of the test, you may get a false negative. Exercising the morning of the test or using laxative medications within a day of the test can also give you a false negative. Some factors can create a false positive too. Smoking the morning of the test, having poor oral hygiene (including dirty dentures), taking probiotic supplements, and having eaten a high-carb dinner or lots of gassy vegetables or beans the evening before may give a false positive. If you are very constipated—or FOS as described in the previous chapter—your breath test may look positive on first glance. A very experienced doctor should be able to detect the subtle differences between a breath gas pattern caused by constipation compared to one actually caused by SIBO, but it's very common for constipated people to receive false-positive diagnoses.

This last point raises the following important issue that affects your SIBO diagnosis: Breath test data are routinely misinterpreted by doctors and other clinicians who aren't very experienced with the condition. Depending on how old your doctor is, he or she may not have learned about breath testing in medical school. And if your doctor uses home-administered tests that you mail away to a lab, then he or she will be relying on the lab to interpret the test results. I've been surprised to see just how inaccurate the interpretations from these labs can be. You should also be aware that alternative medicine providers, functional/integrative doctors, nutritionists, naturopaths, or chiropractors commonly use nonstandard interpretations of the test data that strongly favor positive results for most everyone.

With all of these messy variables, it's no wonder I've seen so many doctors question the usefulness of breath testing to begin with. While I do not share this skepticism, I do think there's an important lesson here for you as a patient: Always request a copy of the breath test data for your records. While the numbers themselves may not mean much to you, they will be extremely helpful to an experienced gastroenterologist or other well-trained health professional who can verify whether you received a proper diagnosis based on the numbers.

Small Bowel Culture

It is possible, but extremely uncommon, for doctors to diagnose SIBO by taking a sample of fluid from your small intestine, culturing it in a lab, and counting how many bacteria are present. This is an invasive and time-consuming process compared to breath testing, so it's generally only done in academic or research environments. In my clinical practice, I've only seen a doctor do this once, and it was for a patient whose SIBO wasn't responding to any of the antibiotics he prescribed. He cultured her small intestinal fluid to see what type of bacteria she was overgrowing so he could tailor the antibiotic choice to her particular critters. If your doctor is planning to examine your small intestine for another reason by doing an endoscopy (see chapter 3 for a refresher), though, it's possible that he or she may piggyback on this procedure and take the fluid sample while in there.

Stool and Blood Tests

SIBO cannot be accurately diagnosed through stool testing or blood tests, so beware of labs that market products or tests that claim otherwise.

Colonoscopy, Endoscopy, and Imaging

SIBO is not visible to the naked eye when a doctor looks at your intestines from the inside through a colonoscopy or an endoscopy, or by examining images of the digestive system with ultrasounds or x-rays. Contrary to popular belief, SIBO is not inflammatory, so there will be no red, inflamed tissue or extra white blood cells even in parts of the intestine affected by SIBO. (However, there may be visible inflammation near the junction of your small intestine and colon that can predispose you to developing SIBO.) One of the few clues to SIBO that doctors may glean from these tests, however, might be an abnormal enlargement of a segment of the small intestine. Such dilation can be caused by too much extra gas in a relatively narrow part of your gastrointestinal tract.

Treating SIBO

There is a pervasive myth that SIBO can never really be treated and that once you have it, you'll keep on getting it. This is not true. While many of my patients with SIBO have had a recurrence at some point after they were treated successfully, this has usually been because their doctor never tried to figure out why they developed the condition to begin with. Remember: SIBO is a symptom of something else. Identifying and correcting the underlying cause makes the possibility of recurrence far less likely. While some underlying causes of SIBO cannot be fixed, plenty of them can be.

I have also come to believe that some of the common advice circulating online may be leading some patients to give themselves SIBO again and again as the result of extensive probiotic supplement regimens—turning a treatable symptom of something else into a chronic condition in and of itself. If you've got a small intestine predisposed to overgrowing (even "good") bacteria, then loading up on concentrated bacteria pills may be doing you more harm than good. Until there is actual scientific evidence that supports the benefit of taking bacterial probiotics in preventing SIBO, I'll continue to caution my patients to steer clear of them entirely. I advise my SIBO patients who wish to take a probiotic to try a yeast-based product called *Florastor;* see chapter 14 for more details.

Medical Treatment for SIBO
Antibiotics
Prescription antibiotics are the only evidence-based treatment for SIBO as of the time of this writing. Many different herbal ingredients are administered in alternative medicine circles as more "natural" sources of antibiotics to treat SIBO; these include oregano oil, berberine, and garlic extract (allicin). However, there is no evidence to support these having an antibiotic effect in the human body (in general) or as being an effective treatment for SIBO in particular. (Most of these haven't been

studied in humans for *any* digestive condition whatsoever, in fact.) See chapter 14 for a more complete discussion of common supplements marketed to treat SIBO and the state of the science surrounding them.

Because SIBO is an overgrowth of the same "good" bacteria you harbor in your colon, any drug that treats the overgrowth will also cause collateral damage to the good bacteria in your colon. Despite some claims you may encounter online, no antibiotics—whether herb-derived or pharmaceutical—are able to target the critters that cause overgrowth but spare the critters that have stayed put in the colon where they belong. They are literally the same organisms, just in a different place. All antibiotics kill their target bacteria indiscriminately. They do not, however, eradicate all of your gut's bacteria completely. Rather, they suppress the total number of bacteria you harbor. Your colon's inner ecosystem usually rebounds to its normal population levels and composition within a month of taking most antibiotics. Cipro (ciprofloxacin) is a notable exception; it takes far longer for your inner ecosystem to rebound from it.

Different antibiotics target different types of organisms that can cause overgrowth. Your doctor should select an antibiotic based on the results of your breath test, which will reveal whether you harbor hydrogen-producing bacteria, methane-producing organisms called *archaea,* or a combination of both. One of the most common antibiotics used to treat SIBO is Xifaxan (rifaxamin). Some doctors may prescribe a cocktail of Xifaxan and another drug if your breath test showed evidence of methane gas. While rifaxamin has a pretty solid track record, not all overgrowing critters respond to it. So if your SIBO symptoms persist after completing a course of this drug, I encourage you to discuss choosing a different antibiotic with your doctor rather than submitting to another course of the same. (Remember the old cliché about insanity? It's defined as doing the same thing over and over and expecting a different result.)

If you live somewhere that is not near a breath-testing facility—or if your doctor is a breath-testing skeptic—then you may be prescribed antibiotics to treat suspected SIBO without actually being tested first. If you're lucky, this will be a shortcut to symptom relief. But there are downsides to consider. If you don't feel better after taking the antibiotics, is it because you don't actually have SIBO or rather because you do have

SIBO but were given an antibiotic mismatched to your particular type? Sometimes doctors who treat SIBO without testing will assume the former instead of the latter and stop pursuing diagnosis and treatment after a failed response to antibiotics.

Dietary Treatment for SIBO

No diet has been scientifically shown to cure SIBO, nor has any diet been shown to prevent you from developing SIBO. If you've been poking around online, you may have encountered competing arguments about whether to restrict your diet at all when you are being treated for SIBO. While many marketers of various diet protocols claim that their diets "starve" bacteria in the gut, these regimens do not actually eradicate SIBO or kill bacteria.

One school of thought argues that you should eat lots and lots of FODMAPs and carbs during treatment to feed the bacteria and "draw them out" so the antibiotics can work most effectively. The opposing school of thought argues you should avoid FODMAPs and carbs during treatment and after as well, in order to "starve" the bacteria, thereby weakening them and preventing risk of recurrence. In reality, there is no scientific evidence to support either argument. Furthermore, both arguments are grounded in a basic misunderstanding of how antibiotics actually work: bacteria don't need to be rapidly multiplying in order to be susceptible to the effects of antibiotics, nor does denying them fermentable carbohydrates weaken them in a manner that would make them more susceptible to these drugs.

From my perspective, the choice as to whether to restrict your diet during treatment for SIBO depends on how miserable you feel symptom-wise and how much of a diet change you're willing to make in order to feel better until the medication works its magic.

Certain diets, however, have been shown to help control the symptoms of untreated SIBO, and they are extremely effective at doing so. In other words, the role of diet when you have SIBO is to help with symptom control until your condition has been successfully treated with medicine.

The two main dietary approaches to SIBO symptom management are described below. No matter which dietary approach you choose from among them, you should be careful of very high-fat foods. High-fat foods may be poorly absorbed when you have SIBO and can worsen symptoms of gas, bloating, and diarrhea.

Low-FODMAP Diet

Doctors and dietitians in Australia developed the low-FODMAP diet as a targeted, science-based elimination diet to help control abdominal pain, excess gas, and irregular bowel patterns. Research studies have shown it to be extremely effective in doing so for people with irritable bowel syndrome (IBS). It's also my diet of choice for patients with SIBO. *FODMAP* is an acronym that refers to several families of carbohydrates that are poorly digested by humans and easily digested by bacteria; the *F* in FODMAP stands for *fermentable*. Some FODMAPs are types of sugar; others are types of starch or fiber.

When you're healthy and you eat foods high in FODMAPs, these carbohydrates nourish the friendly bacteria in your colon and help maintain a healthy, diverse ecosystem in your gut. (You may fart a little bit if you overdo it, but there's no harm in a bit of gas!) But when you've got SIBO and you eat foods high in FODMAPs, these carbohydrates nourish the extra bacterial houseguests you're harboring in your small intestine and can contribute to significant bloating, excessive amounts of gas, and general misery in the bathroom.

The low-FODMAP diet identifies specific foods within each food group that contain high amounts of very fermentable carbohydrates and are likely to trigger symptoms in susceptible people. Unlike many other types of elimination diets, the low-FODMAP diet does not prohibit any entire food groups. There are acceptable fruits, vegetables, grains, nuts, seeds, dairy foods, animal proteins, plant-based proteins, and even sugars on this diet.

While most wheat-containing foods are limited on the low-FODMAP diet, it is not actually a gluten-free diet. In fact, there are some low-FODMAP wheat-containing foods allowed on the diet, and some high-FODMAP gluten-free foods that are prohibited! Similarly, while some dairy foods are limited on the low-FODMAP diet, it is not a dairy-free diet. In fact, there are some low-FODMAP dairy foods allowed and some high-FODMAP dairy-free substitutes that are prohibited! The devil is in the details when it comes to mastering the low-FODMAP diet, so roll up your sleeves and dive into chapter 13 to learn all about it.

Specific Carbohydrate Diet (SCD)

The SCD is a grain-free, low-sugar, low-dairy diet that became popular in the 1980s as a way to manage inflammatory bowel diseases such as Crohn's and colitis. Over the years, many patients have provided testimonials of how the diet helped them either achieve or maintain remission from these digestive diseases. However, there is surprisingly little scientific evidence to support these anecdotes. More recently, the online SIBO community has revived the SCD as a way to manage the gas, bloating, and erratic bowel patterns associated with the condition.

The SCD prohibits all grains; starchy root vegetables such as potatoes, yams, and parsnips; chickpeas and soybeans; most dairy except for hard cheeses and homemade yogurt; and all sugar except for small amounts of honey. As you may have noticed, it's actually quite similar to the more fashionable Paleo diet, except for the allowance of some forms of dairy. It's a pretty low-carbohydrate diet that also happens to eliminate many foods that we now know to be high FODMAP, but it certainly does not eliminate all of them. In this regard, I tend to think of the SCD as version 1.0 of the low-FODMAP diet, invented before we knew why lower carbohydrate diets seemed to ease the symptoms of some people with diarrheal conditions.

The SCD helps many people with SIBO feel better because it inadvertently reduces the FODMAP load of your diet. However, because the SCD still allows high-FODMAP foods, such as honey, fructose-rich fruits, and certain gassier vegetables, people with SIBO may find incomplete symptom relief when on it. In other words, the SCD may be unnecessarily restrictive of some well-tolerated carbs, such as white sugar, maple syrup, rice, and potatoes, and insufficiently restrictive of others, like peas, lentils, pistachios, high-fructose fruits, and vegetables in the cabbage family. I think of the low-FODMAP diet as the nutritional version of a scalpel: a precision diet that removes only the most fermentable carbohydrates that bacteria are able to digest. In contrast, I consider the SCD diet to be the nutritional equivalent of a bludgeon: a heavy-handed solution that may achieve intended results, but whose complete restriction of carbs and sugar in doing so is unnecessarily aggressive. This is why I do not recommend it.

The SIBO Diet

If you've been poking around online, you may have come across the so-called SIBO diet. This regimen generally refers to a hybrid mix of the low-FODMAP and SCD diets. I've found it is unnecessarily restrictive for the vast majority of my patients, who are able to achieve excellent symptom control on the low-FODMAP diet alone. Because it's unnecessarily restrictive for the vast majority of patients I've seen, I do not recommend it.

Elemental Diets

Elemental diets consist of liquid or powdered formulas that have been "predigested" with enzymes so that all the nutrients are broken down into their most basic building blocks. The nutrients in these formulas are absorbed so quickly and completely by your body, there's nothing left for those overgrown bacteria to feast on. Elemental formulas like Nestlé's Vivonex or Abbott's EleCare are medical foods that were originally developed to be fed via a tube directly into the stomachs or intestines of very sick people with severe bowel diseases. If you've ever smelled or tasted one of these formulas, you'd understand why they were not intended to be taken by mouth. Some dietary supplement manufacturers have also begun selling powdered elemental diet formulas that are intended to be somewhat more palatable.

One small study conducted over a decade ago sought to explore whether putting people with SIBO on an elemental diet for two weeks might actually cure SIBO by starving the bacteria. While the results showed promise, this single study was way too short to be conclusive. Many patients had a clean breath test immediately after the elemental diet, but the researchers didn't follow the patients after the initial few weeks of the elemental diet trial to see if their SIBO actually remained at bay after they went off the diet. In other words, due to lack of evidence that elemental diets actually eradicate SIBO for more than a very abbreviated period and the fact that they're seriously difficult to tolerate, I do not recommend them.

Dietary Supplements

If you've encountered the SIBO-industrial-complex online when visiting Dr. Google, then you've probably heard of at least a half dozen supplements that "everyone" recommends for SIBO. There's L-glutamine, oregano oil, garlic extract (allicin), and berberine. Often there's at least one probiotic, a digestive enzyme supplement, and betaine HCl as well. (These common pillars of alternative medicine regimens are discussed in greater detail in chapter 14.) Because these same products are mentioned over and over again in an echo-chamber type of way, it gives the impression that they are standard, well-accepted protocols for treating SIBO. In fact, they are not. No well-designed scientific studies have shown any of these supplements to be of benefit in treating or preventing SIBO (or anything else, for that matter). It's also worth noting the source of these recommendations: many come from websites or practitioners trying to sell you the products in question.

Probiotics

I do want to address the particular question of probiotics when you have SIBO, for two reasons. First, because of the pervasive internet-fueled notion that SIBO results from an imbalance of "good" and "bad" that needs to be rebalanced with probiotic supplements; you might have seen this referred to as *dysbiosis*. I've already dispensed of this myth earlier in this chapter, so suffice it to say I don't consider this a good reason to use probiotics if you have SIBO. Second is that most people choose to treat their SIBO with an antibiotic medication, and there's good evidence that taking certain specific types of probiotics can be beneficial to people who have to use antibiotics for any reason.

Probiotic supplements contain living organisms—either bacteria or yeasts—intended to confer a health benefit on the person taking them. In cases where you need to take an antibiotic, certain probiotics may reduce the common side effect of diarrhea and may also protect you from developing so-called opportunistic infections from disease-causing bacteria when your usual microbial defense system is suppressed by the medication. But here's the rub: If we're trying to kill off all those extra bacteria that your small intestine has decided to overgrow, why on earth would we want to deliver pills full of more bacteria right back into your small intestine?

This is the main reason why I advise against taking any *bacterial* probiotics if you have SIBO or if you've had SIBO in the past and didn't correct the condition that predisposed you to developing it originally. I'm concerned about reseeding a gut predisposed to overgrowing bacteria with pills full of more bacteria. However, not all probiotic supplements are bacteria-based. Some are yeast-based, and these cannot overgrow in the small intestine. Better still: Yeast-based probiotics aren't killed by antibiotic medications, meaning they'll be able to survive the journey to your colon and carry out their health-promoting mission while you're treating your SIBO. Florastor (*Saccharomyces boulardii lyo* CNCM I-745) is a very-well-studied strain of probiotic and the one I recommend for my patients undergoing antibiotic treatment for SIBO. (And for the record, I don't sell it, nor do I have any material relationship with the company.)

Luisa's SIBO Story:
Bloating with a Side of Reflux and Diarrhea

Luisa was a forty-eight-year-old high school teacher who was sent to me by her gastroenterologist for acid reflux disease (GERD). She had recently been put on a proton-pump inhibitor (PPI) medication every morning and an H2 blocker medication at night, which made her feel much better for about a month. But then things started changing for the worse.

For starters, the reflux came back with a vengeance, despite ongoing use of her acid-suppressing medications. She had to give up her nightly glass of wine, which now felt like "swallowing fire." She also gave up coffee, chocolate, tomato sauce, and acidic fruits, but none of it made any difference. Simultaneously, she started having terrible feelings of bloating in her lower abdomen, lots of gas (farting), and a big change in her bathroom habits. Whereas she had tended to run on the constipated side her entire life—having a bowel movement only once every two to three days—suddenly, she was now having four to five bowel movements per day. And they looked strange too. They were very long and thin, very soft, and light in color.

Within minutes of meeting Luisa, I suspected she might

have SIBO. She was certainly at high risk for it, given the combination of her PPI medication and a predisposition to slow motility elsewhere in her GI tract, but it would be up to her doctor to sort that part of it out. A quick trip through her daily dietary habits only strengthened my hunch: her diet was very high in FODMAPs (see chapter 13), and her bloating typically worsened within thirty minutes of eating these meals. She'd wake up feeling fine every day and go to bed in complete agony from reflux, bloating, and gas.

I advised Luisa to go on a low-FODMAP diet for two weeks while she set about scheduling a breath test to rule out SIBO. When I saw her in the office on the morning of the breath test a few weeks later, she mentioned to me that she had been feeling almost 100 percent better on the low-FODMAP diet—the reflux, bloating, and gas were essentially gone, and she was having fewer bowel movements (though they still weren't normal, per se). Sure enough, her test results came back positive for SIBO. A big lesson from Luisa's case is that SIBO often masquerades as other conditions—especially acid reflux disease or irritable bowel syndrome (IBS). However, it often won't respond to the usual remedies that these conditions respond to, nor is it triggered by many of the same foods.

Luisa's doctor called in a prescription for antibiotics before she even left my office, and I advised Luisa to stick to the low-FODMAP diet until she completed her antibiotic regimen. At that point, she should try resuming her normal diet; if she used to tolerate it comfortably before SIBO, she should be able to tolerate it comfortably now that the SIBO was eradicated. I also advised her to avoid taking any bacterial probiotic supplements going forward, as her small bowel seems hospitable to overgrowing even good bacteria. Luisa's doctor took her off the PPI medication that we suspected may have caused the SIBO and put her on a higher dose of the H2 blockers instead. Our goal is to keep Luisa's reflux well controlled through diet, H2 blockers, and, if needed, calcium carbonate antacids for breakthrough symptoms and keep her off PPIs if possible. It's been about a year and a half since I last saw Luisa, and so far, the SIBO has not come back. We're hoping it will stay gone for good!

If your bloating sounded like SIBO, and you got a diagnosis and you're progressing along through your treatment, congratulations! That bloated belly will soon be a distant memory. But some types of bloating resemble certain aspects of SIBO—the toxic-smelling gas, the unbearable gas pain, the urgent, light-colored bowel movements, the "acidic" feeling in your poop—but aren't actually SIBO. Read on to chapter 9, where you'll learn about other potential causes of a gassy gut.

9.

The Gassy Gut: Bloating by Way of Carbohydrate Intolerances

MOST INTESTINAL GAS—WHICH DOCTORS CALL *flatus* but the rest of us know as *farts*—is manufactured by the bacteria that live in our colons. (For those unlucky folks who have too many bacteria living in their small intestines, as described in chapter 8, there will be ample gas produced in that neighborhood as well.) Bacteria only make noticeable amounts of gas when they're well fed, and this process is called *fermentation*. But bacteria can't just feast on anything. The foods they're best able to ferment are various forms of carbohydrates: certain sugars, fibers, or complex starches.

To be clear: Having intestinal gas is not a bad thing, nor is it a sign that something is amiss. Quite the contrary, in fact! Farting is a natural side effect of healthy living when it results from a diet loaded with fiber from healthy foods like beans, veggies, fruits, whole grains, nuts, and seeds. Some of the healthiest people I know are also some of the gassiest. The average person makes anywhere from a half liter to two liters of gas per day and farts eight to twenty times per day.

So when does intestinal gas cross that line from a benign badge of honor from your healthy diet to a harbinger of something digestive gone awry? When it's accompanied by a painful bloated belly, foul odor, diarrhea, being awoken from sleep with an urgent need to defecate, or even incontinence of your feces (pooping accidents). If any of these symptoms sound familiar, you could be dealing with bloating by way of carbohydrate intolerance.

Carbohydrate Intolerances

If you've already read chapter 8, you'll recall that the small intestine is where almost all of our food is broken down into basic nutritional building blocks and absorbed into our bodies for use. If a particular food component doesn't get absorbed in the small intestine, then it continues on its journey toward the colon, where it's greeted by trillions of bacteria. And if the unabsorbed food happens to be easily fermentable by these bacteria, then they'll start feasting on it, producing gas as a by-product. Of all the different types of nutrients we eat, carbohydrates are generally the most easily fermentable by bacteria. In other words, if there's gas in your gut, there's a reasonably good chance it was made by bacteria breaking down some type of carbohydrate.

Our bodies have many different tools for digesting and absorbing the different types of carbohydrates in our diets. We have carb-digesting enzymes, called *amylases*, in the saliva and from the pancreas that break long chains of starch into simple sugars so they can be easily absorbed. We have other enzymes manufactured on the spot by the small intestine's cells themselves, which cleave sugars like lactose (milk sugar) and sucrose (table sugar) into their individual components for easy absorption. We also have dedicated transporters lining the small intestine, whose main job is to shuttle a type of sugar called *fructose* into the intestinal cells.

With all of these digestive tools at your gut's disposal, how might a carbohydrate escape absorption and wind up all the way in your colon as fodder for feasting bacteria? There are several possibilities.

- **LACTOSE INTOLERANCE, OR DEFICIENCY OF THE LACTOSE-DIGESTING ENZYME, LACTASE:** You've probably heard the term *lactose intolerance,* and this is one of the most common types of carbohydrate intolerances around. Lactose intolerance happens when the cells lining your small intestine start producing less and less of the enzyme *lactase,* which is required to break down milk sugar for absorption. If the milk sugar, lactose, can't be cleaved, then it can't be absorbed, so it continues onward toward the colon. Since bacteria can ferment lactose easily, they'll produce lots of gas when they encounter it, and the more lactose they're offered, the more gas they'll make. Large loads of unabsorbed lactose in the colon also attract lots of water through osmosis, so this gas may be accompanied by crampy, urgent diarrhea as well.

  Lactose intolerance is *not* the same as an allergy to dairy or milk. Allergies are inflammatory immune system responses that can affect systems throughout the body. Carbohydrate intolerances are cases of incomplete nutrient absorption that provoke noninflammatory symptoms isolated to the digestive tract. It is not unhealthy or dangerous for lactose-intolerant people to consume foods with lactose . . . just really uncomfortable.

- **FRUCTOSE INTOLERANCE, OR TOO FEW TRANSPORTERS FOR FRUCTOSE SUGARS:** While lactose intolerance is a pretty well-known condition, fewer people have heard of fructose intolerance. But malabsorbing a sugar called *fructose* is relatively common as well—it may affect up to 30 percent of people. Fructose is a sugar that's found naturally in certain fruits and sweeteners like honey and agave nectar. It's also added to foods, candy, and soft drinks in the form of high-fructose corn syrup (HFCS). Our bodies require a special transporter in the small intestine to carry fructose from the digestive tract into the bloodstream. But some people's intestines don't express very many of these transporters—and others simply have poorly functioning transporters. If you're one of these people, you may max out your fructose-absorption capacity with relatively small intakes of this sugar, leaving the excess amounts unabsorbed. The unabsorbed fructose travels on to the colon and provokes the same symptoms of gas, bloating, and diarrhea described above for lactose intolerance.

- **CONSUMING INDIGESTIBLE SUGAR ALCOHOLS (POLYOLS):** While our bodies have different ways to absorb a variety of sugars, there's a cousin of sugar that humans have minimal capacity to absorb. This cousin is called a *sugar alcohol* or *polyol,* and it's similar enough to sugar in structure to taste sweet, but not similar enough to piggyback on sugar's digestive pathways. Different types of sugar alcohols are found naturally in certain fruits and vegetables like prunes, cauliflower, and avocados. They're also added to sugar-free foods, drinks, gums, candies, medications, and supplements to help provide sweet taste without lots of calories or the risk of promoting dental caries. After all, if you can't absorb sugar alcohols, then they can't provide much by way of calories!

  You'll recognize sugar alcohols on a food label as anything that ends with the suffix -*ol*: sorbitol, xylitol, mannitol, erythritol, lactitol. Because sugar alcohols aren't absorbed in the small intestine, they travel on to the colon and are available for fermentation by the resident bacteria. When they arrive in higher doses, they can provoke the same symptoms of gas, bloating, and diarrhea described in the sections above on lactose and fructose intolerance. In fact, some sugar alcohols are deliberately marketed as laxatives! The sugar alcohol sorbitol is largely responsible for the well-known laxative effect of prunes.

- **EATING FERMENTABLE FIBERS FROM PLANT FOODS:** If you've ever noticed the remnants of corn kernels in your poop, then you get the basic gist of fiber; it is, by definition, not digestible to human beings. Fiber describes any type of carbohydrate from plant foods that humans lack the digestive enzymes to break down. Our inability to break down these plant food components—fruit, vegetable, and bean skins; bran from whole grains; seed coatings; and all those stringy bits in leafy veggies, pineapple, and celery—is actually what makes them so beneficial to our health. (Chapter 11 includes a fuller discussion about the health benefits of fiber.)

  But while fiber is indigestible to us humans, much of it is very digestible to all those bacteria that live in our colons, and when they encounter their favorite types of fiber, they may produce a fair amount of gas to show you their appreciation. The amount of gas produced varies based on the type of fiber, as some types are more fermentable than others. Very fermentable types of fiber are called *high FODMAP*; you can read more about them in chapter 13. The amount of gas produced by type of fiber will also vary among people, as it depends to some extent on what type of bacteria you happen to harbor.

Even if you were to make the same exact amount of gas as your friend with a gut of steel, there's no guarantee that it would affect you the same way. One person may hardly notice the gas they produce following a bowl of black beans and broccoli; someone else may find themselves in agony for days. In other words, no human being can digest fiber, so it's perfectly normal to produce gas when you eat it. But foods rich in fermentable fibers are only a problem for you if they're a problem for you. The gas itself is benign; the gas pains and bloating you may experience because of it, however, may be a problem you need to reckon with.

Gas from all of these carbohydrate intolerances generally kicks in about six to eight hours after you consume the offending carb, though in some cases it can start as early as four hours. As mentioned above, if you don't absorb lactose, fructose, or sugar alcohols but consume a particularly large portion of them, you may also experience diarrhea. If the dose is extra-extra-large, you could wake up overnight with urgent diarrhea or even have an episode of fecal incontinence (a pooping accident). As unpleasant as their symptoms are, though, carbohydrate intolerances aren't at all harmful to your health. The diarrhea they provoke is not inflammatory, and it does not do any damage to the gut itself.

Some carbohydrate intolerances can happen naturally on their own, while others can be a temporary result of another medical condition. For example, you may be genetically programmed to produce less lactase enzyme as you age, which causes you to become lactose intolerant in later childhood, adolescence, or your twenties. Alternatively, you may be programmed to produce plenty of lactase enzyme well into adulthood, but you happen to damage the cells in your small intestines that produce lactase enzyme. This damage may result from the onset of celiac disease (see chapter 10) or even just a nasty diarrheal infection. In these latter cases, you may experience temporary lactose intolerance that can improve once the damaged small intestinal lining has had time to repair itself.

If you happen to notice that multiple different carb-containing foods—including dairy foods with lactose, fruits and treats with fructose, a variety of vegetables, wheat, and/or beans—have suddenly started provoking bad gas and bloating seemingly out of nowhere, you might consider the possibility of SIBO (see chapter 8). The type of carbohydrate intolerances caused by SIBO are temporary, and any foods you were able to eat comfortably before you had the condition should be comfortably tolerated again once you complete successful antibiotic treatment. Gas and bloating from SIBO typically sets in much faster than gas and bloating from other carbohydrate intolerances—usually within sixty to ninety minutes of eating the offending carbs.

What Bloating from Carbohydrate Intolerances Feels Like

Bloating from carbohydrate intolerance is inevitably accompanied by lots of gas, primarily the farting kind rather than the belching kind. The gas is often quite smelly; my patients commonly describe it as "toxic"; others have employed more colorful nicknames, like *green smoke* or *death farts*. While gas produced through the normal course of digestive business may prompt you to fart once or twice over the course of a few hours, gas from carb malabsorption typically comes in unrelenting attacks that involve near-constant farting for an hour or more as the unabsorbed carb arrives to the colon and is greeted by hungry masses of bacteria.

Gas and bloating attacks will often set in immediately after eating a meal, but the tricky thing is that it's not the meal you just ate that caused the gas attack but rather something you ate one or two meals prior. For example, if you are fructose intolerant and ate honey and mango for breakfast, you may start to feel gassy and bloated immediately after finishing lunch. The act of eating lunch triggers your gastrocolic reflex (described in chapter 7, page 93) and propels the previous meal forward in the colon, where the consequences of malabsorption make themselves known.

Bloating from unabsorbed carbohydrates may feel like your belly is "inflated" full of gas, but even constant farting seems to do nothing to alleviate it. A doctor examining your belly may find it to be taut like a drum. You may hear gas swishing and gurgling around in the part of your gut below your belly button. Sometimes you may not feel your belly can become flat again until you "reset" overnight in your sleep (when you may fart unabashedly).

Bloating from malabsorption can also be quite painful, and the pain derives from gas pressure. (If bloating is accompanied by diarrhea, it will often include some crampy pain as well.) Some people experience gas pressure as sharp pains in the center to lower part of the abdomen, while others sometimes feel the gas pain radiating to their sides or back. It's sometimes the kind of gas pain that makes my patients feel the need to lie down and curl up into a ball. Taking anti-gas remedies like Gas-X or Phazyme (simethicone) does nothing to alleviate this type of bloating and gas pain once it has set in; it's too little too late.

Looser stools, urgent bowel movements, or overt diarrhea often accompany bloating from malabsorption of lactose, fructose, or sugar alcohols. The diarrhea you get from carbohydrate intolerances is the kind that might wake you from sleep early in the morning or be so urgent as to cause an accident. The stool may be lighter colored than usual—more orangey brown—and it may feel a bit "acidic" on its way out. You may also experience an itchy anus after passing one of these stools. For real-life testimonials as to the crampy, urgent, laxative effect of sugar alcohols in particular, go online and read through some of the customer reviews for sugar-free gummy bears on Amazon.com. Doing so may bring some needed comic relief to your very uncomfortable situation.

Diagnosing Carbohydrate Intolerances

Breath Testing

Breath testing is a safe, noninvasive, painless way to check whether you malabsorb lactose or fructose. (It can also be used to diagnose SIBO; see chapter 8 for more details.) Human cells cannot produce hydrogen or methane gas, but bacteria can. So doctors can check your breath for traces of these gases after you've been given a drink sweetened with either lactose or fructose. If you absorb the sugar fully, no increase in these gases should be detectable on your breath. If you don't absorb the sugar, then the telltale evidence of bacterial fermentation—hydrogen or methane gas—should begin to appear on your breath between two and three hours after drinking the solution.

The test involves showing up at a doctor's office first thing in the morning, fasted. You'll breathe into a bag and then drink a solution sweetened with 25 grams of lactose or fructose—the rough equivalent of two glasses of milk or a twelve-ounce can of Coca-Cola, respectively. Then, every fifteen to thirty minutes for the next three hours, you'll breathe into a bag. Your exhaled breath captured in the bag will be fed into a machine that measures the types of gases it contains. If the hydrogen or methane on your breath increases more than a prescribed amount from that initial measurement, you'll be diagnosed with lactose or fructose intolerance.

Unfortunately, doctors are not very experienced in interpreting hydrogen breath test results. For this reason, I always encourage my patients to obtain copies of their breath test results—the actual numbers recorded from each breath—so that I can double-check them along with other members of their care team. The particular concern is that when you're being tested for lactose or fructose intolerance, the results may provide clues that suggest you actually have SIBO instead. An experienced clinician will be able to tell the difference between the conditions based on when the gases on your breath begin to rise.

Blood Testing

Blood testing is a far less precise way to measure lactose intolerance and is scarcely used since the advent of breath tests. Few doctors employ it anymore. Other blood tests that purport to measure food intolerances or food sensitivities lack scientific evidence. Common tests include those which measure IgG antibodies to various foods, so-called MRT testing and Alcat food sensitivity testing. I do not recommend using these expensive and unproven approaches.

Elimination Diets/Food Challenges

While we have objective ways to diagnose lactose and fructose intolerance (the breath tests described above), there are no reliable, scientifically validated ways to objectively test for intolerance to other carbohydrates. In theory, everyone should malabsorb sugar alcohols and fiber, so there's really no point in even testing for it. However, if you're trying to identify whether consuming sugar alcohols or a particular type of fiber is responsible for your bloating and distress, then an elimination diet is my preferred approach.

You can approach elimination diets in a targeted way or in a broad way. As a trained dietitian, I can often come up with a pretty good guess as to the most likely culprit of your gas and bloating based on the timing of your symptom onset relative to the timing and content of your previous meals. For example, if your gas and bloating kick in at 3:00 P.M. like clockwork, I'll be looking to see what high-FODMAP foods or drinks you consumed six to eight hours earlier, at 7:00–9:00 A.M. Based on the hypothesis I generate from this dietary detective work, I may advise you to only eliminate that particular food or ingredient. This targeted approach to elimination dieting often gets to an answer faster and without too much disruption to your daily diet.

Sometimes, though, a single gas and bloating trigger is harder to identify. This is the case for my patients whose frequency of gas and bloating is more erratic, whose diets are not consistent at all, or whose diets are so loaded with multiple kinds of FODMAPs that it's difficult to isolate the effect of any one particular food. In these cases, a more encompassing elimination diet is warranted, and I'll often recommend a two-week FODMAP-elimination diet. (Chapter 13 will describe this protocol in detail.) In the vast majority of cases, the gas and bloating resolve during this period (and when they don't, that itself is a clue as well). Then we can challenge one type of FODMAP at a time to see which types of carbohydrates are most responsible for provoking the gas and bloating.

I'm aware that many other types of elimination diets are quite common, and their protocols involve some combination of gluten-free, grain-free, dairy-free, sugar-free, soy-free, yeast-free, and nightshade-free. In my experience, these far-ranging protocols impose a huge burden on a person. Even when they produce good results, it can take ages to help you figure out which of the dozens of eliminated items was actually problematic. In other words, this approach tends not to be specific enough to pinpoint exactly what the offending food item(s) is/are. When you eventually tire of the excessively restricted protocol and abandon it entirely, you're none the wiser as to what was troubling you than you were when you started.

For example, your gas and bloating may resolve on an everything-free diet, but does that tell you whether eliminating dairy was what made a difference? And if you do realize that eliminating dairy was what helped, was it because you're lactose intolerant? If so, you needn't have eliminated *all* dairy . . . just all lactose-containing dairy. (And a breath test could have gotten you this answer without having to eliminate anything!) But chances are, once you've felt better on a fully dairy-free diet, you aren't going back—and you're stuck with a diet restriction that may be overkill for your needs.

Similarly, if your gas and bloating resolve on a gluten-free diet (and your doctor has already ruled out celiac disease), is it really because you have a digestive intolerance to gluten—the *protein* in wheat? Or is it because you're reacting badly to the fermentable *carbohydrate* in wheat, which is a type of FODMAP called a *fructan*? This distinction has major implications: If you mistakenly believe yourself to be gluten intolerant, you'll spend the rest of your life fretting unnecessarily about minute amounts of cross-contamination at restaurants. If you figure out that you simply have a digestive disagreement with the carbohydrates in wheat, you'll realize that you can tolerate some forms of wheat-based foods just fine—like sourdough bread—and that there's no need for you to worry about foods with trace amounts of gluten, like conventional oatmeal, soy sauce, or cross-contaminated restaurant foods.

Treating Carbohydrate Intolerances

Medical Treatment for Carbohydrate Intolerances

Since carbohydrate intolerances are not harmful to your health, there is no need to seek medical treatment for them. You can manage symptoms by avoiding trigger foods. If you love a particular carbohydrate that doesn't love you back, though, you can try using specific enzyme supplements (when available) to improve digestibility of the offending food.

Over-the-Counter Enzyme Supplements

Over-the-counter lactase enzyme supplements are available to prevent lactose malabsorption if you're lactose intolerant and want to continue eating high-lactose dairy foods. When taken right with the first bite of a lactose-containing meal, lactase supplements should enable you to absorb the lactose in your meal without the usual consequences. Lactase supplements are marketed under the Lactaid and Dairy Ease brand names, but generic store brands are also widely available. Be aware that many "fast-acting" chewable tablet forms of lactase contain sugar alcohols as a filler ingredient and can be gassy in their own right! Read the ingredient labels and choose products that don't contain any inactive ingredients ending with the suffix *-ol*.

More recently, an enzyme supplement called *xylose isomerase* has hit the market, promising to do for fructose intolerance what lactase has done for lactose intolerance. The enzyme reportedly works by promoting a chemical reaction that transforms fructose into another, more digestible sugar: glucose. The science behind this product seems pretty sound, though because it's relatively new to market, I haven't had too many patients try it and verify that it works as intended. See chapter 14 for a more detailed discussion.

Another enzyme—which can help with gas and bloating caused by malabsorption of a particular type of FODMAP found in beans, veggies in the cabbage family, and even some nuts—is alpha-galactosidase. It is marketed as Beano, Bean-zyme, and in generic store-brand versions as well. Alpha-galactosidase is an enzyme borrowed from a type of mold that has the ability to digest complex fibers that mammals don't.

When you take it with the first bites of a meal that contains these fibers—whether from beans, broccoli, brussels sprouts, or pistachio nuts—the fiber can be broken down and absorbed in your small intestine. (See chapter 13, page 202, for a full list of foods with this type of fiber, called *galacto-oligosaccharides*, or GOS.) Therefore, these typically gassy foods should not contribute to very much gas in the colon. Just as many lactase enzyme supplements contain sugar alcohols like mannitol as a filler ingredient, so too is the case for alpha-galactosidase supplements. Read the ingredient labels and choose products that don't contain any inactive ingredients ending with the suffix *-ol*.

Enzymes derived from fruit, like papayas (papain) and pineapples (bromelain), are *not* effective for carbohydrate intolerances. What makes something an enzyme is that it enables a *specific* chemical reaction. Fruit-derived enzymes digest proteins, not sugars or carbs. In other words, neither papain nor bromelain are able to split apart a lactose molecule, transform fructose into something more digestible, or break down gassy vegetable fibers.

Other multidigestive enzyme supplements, which can contain up to a dozen different enzymes, are also quite popular. Typically, these products contain lactase (for lactose digestion) and alpha-galactosidase (for bean and certain veggie fiber digestion), in addition to various types of starch-, protein-, and fat-digesting enzymes that your well-functioning pancreas makes plenty of. In other words, if the source of your gas and bloating is lactose or veggie fiber malabsorption, these products may help. But you're also paying extra for a lot of "bonus" enzymes that don't help; taking more of something you already have doesn't provide any benefit.

Dietary Treatment for Carbohydrate Intolerances

If malabsorbing a particular carbohydrate is the source of your woes, then the dietary remedy is simple: Stop eating it. Still, if you choose to throw caution to the wind, your reaction will depend on the dose you consumed; eating a little bit of your trigger carb will give you a little bit of gas and bloating, while eating a lot of it will produce a lot of gas and bloating (and in some cases, diarrhea too). For this reason, some people find they can get away with small portions of a food without paying too heavy a price. Trial and error is the only way to figure out what you can get away with.

It's very common for people who are digestively sensitive to fructose to be sensitive to sugar alcohols also. If some allowed fruits on the low-fructose list still seem to bother you, I'd suggest trying to avoid those that contain sugar alcohols as well, listed on page 133 in table 9.2.

TABLE 9.1: Low-Lactose Diet for Lactose Intolerance

	High-Lactose Foods (best to avoid)	Moderate-Lactose Foods (watch portions)	Low-Lactose/ Lactose-Free Foods (eat freely)
Beverages / Liquids	Milk (cow's, goat's and sheep's) Hot cocoa mix Buttermilk Lattes Cappuccinos Egg Nog	Yogurt drinks and dairy-based kefirs	Lactose-free milk Almond milk, soy milk, coconut milk, and other plant-based "milks"
Protein Foods	Ricotta cheese Paneer (Indian cottage cheese) Whey protein concentrate (protein powder and energy bar additive)	Cottage cheese Greek yogurt Regular yogurt Goat's and sheep's milk yogurt Mozzarella cheese Milk protein concentrate	Lactose-free dairy yogurt Nondairy/vegan yogurts made from almond, coconut, or soy milk Hard/aged cheeses, such as cheddar, swiss, Parmesan, feta, American Whey protein isolate (protein powder and energy bar additive)
Desserts / Sweets	Ice cream Milkshakes Gelato Frozen yogurt Custards, including crème brûlée, flan, crème caramel, panna cotta Pudding, rice pudding Dulce de leche Cheesecake Tres leches cake Fudge Anything made with condensed milk (e.g., pumpkin pies, Vietnamese coffee)	Milk chocolate Sherbet	Lactose-free ice cream Nondairy frozen treats (sorbet, vegan "ice cream")
Ingredi-ents / Misc.	Evaporated/condensed milk Lactose (used in medicine as a filler or milk chocolate candy bars)	Whipped cream (larger potions)	Half and half Butter Cream cheese

TABLE 9.2: Low-Fructose Diet for Fructose Intolerance

	High in Fructose (avoid)	Low in Fructose (should be safe)
Beverages/ Liquids	Soda made with high-fructose corn syrup (HFCS) Sports drinks or energy gels/shots made with fructose or HFCS Iced teas and soft drinks made with HFCS Fortified wines (sherry, port) Apple juice and cider Cranberry juice cocktail Most other fruit juices (including cocktail mixers!) Smoothies made with juice base or high-fructose fruits Green juices made with apple as a base Bloody Mary mixes made with HFCS	Natural/"Mexican" sodas made with real sugar Soft drinks or sports drinks sweetened with sugar or glucose 100% cranberry juice (sweetened with sugar) Lemonade sweetened with sugar Regular wine and champagne Unsweetened tea and iced tea
Fruit/ Veggies	Apples/applesauce Cherries Figs Mangoes Pears Watermelon Asparagus	Bananas (ripe but firm is best) Berries Cantaloupe Citrus fruits (oranges, grapefruit, clementines, tangerines, lemons, limes) Grapes Honeydew Kiwis Papayas Pineapples
Sweeteners/ Ingredients	Honey Agave nectar High-fructose corn syrup (HFCS) Fructose Fruit juice concentrates (e.g., pear, apple, grape, etc.) Molasses Invert sugar	White sugar (a.k.a. sugar, table sugar, sucrose, dextrose, evaporated cane syrup) Brown sugar 100% maple syrup Brown rice syrup Glucose syrup Corn syrup Artificial sweeteners (all) Stevia

continued

	High in Fructose (avoid)	Low in Fructose (should be safe)
Condiments	"Pancake syrup"	100% maple syrup
	Ketchup made with HFCS	Organic ketchup made with sugar
	Relishes made with HFCS	
	Tomato sauces made with HFCS	Tomato sauce with no added sugar
	Salad dressings and marinades made with HFCS	Mustard
	BBQ sauces made with honey	Mayonnaise
	Jams/jellies made with fruits or sweeteners listed above	Soy sauce
		Herbs and spices
	Mango or other fruit chutneys	Vinegars
		Oils
		Butter
		Berry jams/jellies or orange marmalade sweetened with real sugar
Desserts/ Sweets	Many "80 calorie" yogurts	Berry, lemon, or coconut sorbet
	Fruit leathers	Premium ice cream sweetened with sugar
	Gummy candies, fruit chews	
	Caramels	Homemade or commercial baked goods sweetened with sugar
	Honey-containing desserts, such as baklava	
	Honey-containing granolas and granola bars	
	Commercial baked goods made with HFCS	
	Fruit pastries, danishes, and pies	
	Fruit compotes	

TABLE 9.3: Foods to Avoid with Sugar Alcohol/Polyol Intolerance

	High in Sugar Alcohols/ Polyols (avoid)	Low in Sugar Alcohols/ Polyols (safe)
Fruit and Juices (and desserts, bars and snacks made with them)	Avocados Apples (and applesauce) Apricots Blackberries Cherries Lychees Peaches Pears Plums Watermelon Dried fruit (prunes, apricots, etc.) Apple juice Tart cherry juice Cranberry juice cocktail Green juices and smoothies made with apple as a base Prune juice Pear and apricot nectar/juice Reduced-calorie/diet juices	Bananas Blueberries Cantaloupe Citrus fruits (oranges, grapefruit, clementines, tangerines, lemons, limes) Figs Grapes Kiwis Honeydew Mangoes Papayas Pineapples Raspberries Strawberries 100% cranberry juice Lemonade sweetened with real sugar
Vegetables	Cauliflower Celery Mushrooms Snow peas Sugar snap peas	All others not listed
Sweeteners/ Ingredients	Sorbitol Xylitol Mannitol Erythritol Lactitol Truvia (contains erythritol)	Aspartame Agave Honey 100% maple syrup Saccharin Stevia Sucralose (Splenda) Sugar

continued

	High in Sugar Alcohols/ Polyols (avoid)	Low in Sugar Alcohols/ Polyols (safe)
Other/Misc.	Sugarless gum, mints, and candy	All others not forbidden
	Sugar-free chocolates, cookies, and cakes	
	No-sugar-added, sugar-free, and reduced-calorie frozen yogurt, ice cream, and popsicles	
	Some diet/low-calorie sodas, soft drinks, iced teas	
	Some low-carb/low-sugar bars	
	Some sugar-free jellies and jams	
	Sugar-free pancake syrup	
	Kids'/chewable vitamins and sublingual vitamin B_{12} supplements	

10.

Malabsorptive Bloating: Celiac Disease and Pancreatic Insufficiency

THIS CHAPTER IS SOMEWHAT DIFFERENT from the others in the book, as it describes two *organic diseases*. Organic diseases are those caused by physical changes to organs or tissues in your body, rather than by problems with how your apparently normal abdominal muscles, nerves, and organs are functioning. Both of these diseases cause malabsorption and result in bloating as a side effect, though bloating is rarely the only—and is not the most serious—symptom. The conditions are celiac disease and pancreatic insufficiency (PI).

The carbohydrate intolerances described in the previous chapter are the most common causes of bloating by malabsorption and are harmless, albeit uncomfortable. Unlike medically benign carbohydrate intolerances like lactose intolerance or fructose intolerance, however, celiac disease and pancreatic insufficiency can result in severe nutritional deficiencies and significant weight loss.

Pancreatic Insufficiency (PI)

Your pancreas is an organ that produces many of the enzymes your body needs to break down starches, proteins, and fats for absorption. It delivers all of these enzymes to your small intestine, on demand, when food starts arriving there from the stomach. But if the pancreas isn't able to manufacture or deliver enough of these enzymes to cover your digestive needs, you may malabsorb any or all types of nutrients: carbohydrates, proteins, and/or fat. Pancreatic insufficiency describes the condition where you have an abnormally low production or impaired release of digestive enzymes by your pancreas. It's more common among elderly people and people with alcoholism than among younger people and teetotalers. Certain other medical disorders are a risk factor for pancreatic insufficiency, including a past history of acute pancreatitis (inflamed pancreas) and cystic fibrosis.

What Bloating from PI Feels Like

Bloating from PI results in lots of gas and is usually accompanied by large volumes of foul-smelling diarrhea, lower-abdominal cramping (under your belly button), and floating, pale-colored stools that may appear oily. Your poop may be hard to flush, as its greasy texture sticks to the sides of the toilet bowl. You may also be found to be deficient in certain vitamins and will probably also lose a noticeable amount of weight without meaning to do so; this is the result of malabsorbing significant amounts of the calories you consume. If you have symptoms of PI, visit your doctor for further investigation promptly; it can be a clue to a more serious underlying medical problem. With PI, it's actually the fat malabsorption that causes the worst of your gas, bloating, and diarrhea symptoms.

Diagnosing Pancreatic Insufficiency

Stool Testing

PI is generally diagnosed by having a lab analyze a stool sample you provide. A stool test called a *fecal elastase test* measures the amount of an enzyme called *elastase* in your stool and compares it to a normal standard. The well-accepted standard of what's considered normal is anything above 200 micrograms of elastase per gram of stool; levels below this are indicative of PI.

If you're under the care of an alternative medicine practitioner or integrative doctor, be aware that they may send your stool to labs that define normal elastase levels at a much higher threshold. This typically results in overdiagnosis of PI and recommendations to take extensive, expensive regimens of over-the-counter digestive enzyme supplements and animal-derived bile supplements that may be medically unnecessary.

A seventy-two-hour fecal fat test is another stool test that measures the amount of fat in your stool over a three-day period when you are consuming a very high-fat diet. As this description suggests, it's pretty cumbersome to undergo: You'll need to collect your stool for three days, storing it in the fridge as you go, and bring it to the lab for analysis. The fecal fat test is used to determine whether you are malabsorbing fat, but it is less specific than the fecal elastase test in terms of diagnosing PI. (There are other reasons a person could malabsorb fat besides PI.) However, if your fecal fat test is normal, it's pretty unlikely that you have PI.

Medical Treatment for Pancreatic Insufficiency
Pancreatic Enzyme Replacement Therapy (PERT)
When the pancreas cannot deliver enough digestive enzymes to ensure you absorb all of your nutrients, then you'll need to take prescription pancreatic enzyme pills with every meal and snack other than those made of pure sugar, like candy or soda. These prescription enzymes are very different from over-the-counter dietary supplements marketed as digestive enzymes.

For starters, many prescription enzymes are coated in a particular way to ensure they are protected when passing through the acidic stomach to arrive intact to your small intestine. These enzymes only work in a relatively more alkaline environment like the small bowel; if they're cheaply coated (or uncoated), they'll just be digested in the stomach along with your food and rendered inactive. Secondly, prescription enzymes come in standardized and precise doses based on how much of the fat-digesting enzyme, lipase, they contain. This ensures that you can maintain consistent symptom control once you settle on the dose that works best for you. Over-the-counter digestive enzymes marketed as dietary supplements are poorly regulated, unstandardized, and untested for safety and efficacy. They have much lower levels of lipase, and they may or may not be properly coated to resist digestion in the stomach. For these reasons, they are a poor substitute for PERT when you're dealing with a relatively serious condition like PI.

Lastly, prescription PERT is likely to be covered by insurance as a medication; over-the-counter dietary supplements will not be. In the United States, there are six brands of PERT that are approved by the Food and Drug Administration: Creon, Zenpep, Pancreaze, Ultresa, Viokase, and Pertyze.

Dietary Treatments for Pancreatic Insufficiency

In addition to taking your PERT consistently with all meals and snacks that contain nutrients beyond just sugar, there are other dietary approaches to consider as well.

Supplement Water-Soluble Versions of Vitamins A, D, E, and K

Four of the many vitamins our bodies require are considered *fat soluble*, which means they can only be absorbed along with fat. This poses a problem for people with PI who have an impaired ability to absorb fat, as it can lead to deficiencies in these essential nutrients. To address this problem, pharmaceutical companies have developed modified versions of vitamins A, D, E, and K that are *water soluble:* they do not require fat for absorption. Two such products are marketed under the names AquADEKs and DEKAs, respectively, here in the United States. They are available over the counter. Some pharmaceutical companies who market PERT even offer customer loyalty programs that provide free water-soluble vitamin supplements.

Stop Drinking Alcohol

A leading cause of PI is alcohol abuse. Even if your PI wasn't caused by excess alcohol intake, the fact remains that drinking alcohol will only worsen an inflamed, impaired pancreas. There are very few stronger arguments for giving up alcohol than a diagnosis of PI.

Include Easy-to-Digest Starchy Foods and Sugars in your Diet

Our digestive system was designed to have multiple, overlapping tools to digest carbohydrates in our diets. While our pancreatic enzymes do most of the digestive heavy lifting, we still produce other enzymes in the saliva and in the small intestine that can digest simple sugars and low-fat, simple starches like white bread, white rice, refined corn, and potatoes. For this reason, if you have PI, you may be able to digest and absorb these foods more easily than foods high in protein and fat that rely more heavily on the pancreatic enzymes for digestion, causing less bloating and diarrhea and helping you to stabilize your weight if needed. Examples include low-fiber breakfast cereals (like Rice Krispies, Special K, Corn Flakes, Chex, Crispix, Kix), cooked cereals (like cream of wheat/farina, grits, cream of rice), baked potatoes, toast with jam, rice cakes, cooked rice, and fruit juice.

Also, be sure to take your time chewing; this will allow maximum exposure to the digestive enzymes in your saliva before swallowing so that more of your food will arrive "predigested" to your intestines.

Celiac Disease

Celiac disease is an autoimmune disease where your body's immune cells are provoked into attacking the lining of your small intestine. This causes inflammation and damages the intestine's ability to absorb key vitamins, minerals, and sometimes even food energy itself. This self-directed attack is triggered when affected people consume a protein in wheat, barley, and rye called *gluten*. If you have celiac disease, the inflammatory immune response quiets down when you strictly and consistently avoid foods that contain gluten or that have been contaminated with even trace amounts of gluten through cross contact during processing or cooking. The small intestine's lining eventually heals if you strictly avoid eating gluten permanently, and its ability to absorb nutrients is restored to normal.

There are many different ways that celiac disease announces itself, and not all of them involve digestive symptoms. In fact, some people with celiac disease don't experience any bloating, gas, or change in bathroom habits at all—at least not in the early stages of the disease. In these cases, your doctor may think to test for celiac based on a signature skin rash you develop; an unexplained finding of iron deficiency anemia; having osteoporosis or low bone-mineral density at an unusually young age; or because you've lost quite a bit of weight without trying to. This is sometimes called *silent celiac disease*.

What Bloating from Celiac Disease Feels Like

In addition to (or instead of) any of the non-digestive symptoms listed above, if you are among the majority of people with celiac disease who do experience digestive symptoms, then you may find yourself with a type of bloating that feels like your belly "blows up" like a balloon after eating foods that contain gluten: bread, pasta, cereal, baked goods made with flour, pretzels, and many, many others. It is generally a very visible, pregnant-looking bloat, and it may take up to several days to deflate after eating the offending gluten-containing food. (This is different from bloating from carbohydrate intolerances, which usually deflates overnight while you sleep.) As a result of the increase in your abdominal girth, you may not be able to button your pants.

Bloating from celiac disease is often accompanied by generalized abdominal pain—patients describe it as feeling like they always have a stomachache—and significant amounts of gas (farting). The gas can often smell particularly bad; I've had patients describe it as "barnyard" smelling and like "toxic waste." Diarrhea is even more common than bloating among people with celiac disease; it is actually the most common symptom of the disease. A small minority of people do not experience diarrhea, though, and it's not unheard of to experience constipation instead.

Diagnosing Celiac Disease

If you suspect you may have celiac disease, it's important to keep eating at least some gluten regularly until your doctor can complete the necessary diagnostic tests. If you undergo these tests when you have been gluten-free for a few weeks already, there is a strong possibility of receiving a false negative.

Blood Antibody Testing

The first step to diagnosing celiac disease is by checking your blood for an antibody called *tissue transglutaminase,* or *tTg-IgA,* which indicates the presence of an autoimmune attack. Your doctor will also check for your total amount of antibodies (total IgA) to ensure that your immune system is competent enough to produce a reliable test result; a small minority of people have a deficiency in IgA antibodies that make a false negative possible. The tTg antibody is the most reliable marker for celiac disease and will be positive for 98 percent of people with celiac disease. However, it is not entirely specific to celiac disease and can be high for people with other autoimmune diseases too.

Your doctor will also likely check your blood for other antibodies called *deamidated gliadin peptide IgA* and *IgG antibodies* (DGP IgA and IgG). These are used to prevent false negative results. Specifically, they can be helpful to identify potential celiac disease in people who have an IgA deficiency or who fall into that 2 percent minority of folks with celiac disease who do not have a positive tTg antibody test.

Endoscopy (EGD)

If any of the blood antibody tests come back high, then your doctor will likely proceed with phase two of the diagnostic process: an endoscopy. Endoscopy is a procedure done under sedation, where a gastroenterologist sends a camera down your esophagus, through your stomach, and into your small intestine to gather some tissue samples. These biopsies are examined under a microscope for the telltale signs of celiac disease. Based on the results of your blood tests combined with your endoscopy, a doctor can diagnose celiac disease.

Skin Rash Biopsy

Some people with celiac disease may develop an itchy, signature rash that resembles eczema and often clusters on the elbows, knees, back, and buttocks; it is called *dermatitis herpetiformis* (DH). A dermatologist may take a biopsy (tissue sample) of the skin directly next to the lesion and send it to a lab for examination. If the lab finds evidence of IgA antibodies in the skin sample, you may be diagnosed with celiac disease without having to undergo an endoscopy—though your dermatologist may still refer you to a gastroenterologist to confirm the diagnosis. Some people with DH may never experience bloating, diarrhea, or other digestive system complaints as a result of their celiac disease even if their gut is inflamed and malabsorption is occurring. Following a strict gluten-free diet will, however, keep the rash away and ensure your intestines remain healthy and functional for the long term.

Gene Testing (Blood)

It is increasingly common for people with a long history of digestive problems to arrive at our office on a self-prescribed gluten-free diet, making it impossible to verify a diagnosis of celiac disease through blood tests and endoscopy. In such cases, a blood test that checks for the presence of the two gene types associated with celiac disease can help us determine whether celiac disease is even a possibility. People who do not have either the HLA-DQ2 or HLA-DQ8 genes are extremely unlikely to have celiac disease. If you have neither gene, there's a greater than 99 percent chance you won't develop celiac disease. In other words, a negative test means your doctor can almost certainly rule out the possibility of celiac disease.

However, gene testing cannot reveal whether you *do* have celiac disease. This is because 25–30 percent of all Americans carry at least one of these genes, but only about 1 percent of the population will ever go on to develop celiac disease. If you do test positive for one or both of these genes, all it tells us is that we cannot exclude the possibility of your having celiac disease. In fact, if you've been strictly gluten-free for a long period of time and are still experiencing gas, bloating, and/or diarrhea, it's pretty likely that your symptoms are *not* being caused by celiac disease or gluten. As I tell my patients, it can't be bothering you if you're not actually eating it!

Treating Celiac Disease

Medical Treatments for Celiac Disease

The medical treatment for celiac disease is the same as the dietary one: a strict, gluten-free diet for life. *There are no medications or supplements that can reverse celiac disease or enable safe gluten consumption in people with celiac disease.* While some supplement companies market an over-the-counter enzyme called *DPP-IV* (*dipeptidyl peptidase IV*), or *glutenase,* that they claim helps to digest gluten, these are not effective for people with celiac disease and do not make gluten safe to eat if you have celiac.

Dietary Treatment for Celiac Disease

At present, a strict, gluten-free (GF) diet is the only effective treatment for the symptoms of celiac disease. Following a strict gluten-free diet enables your gut to heal completely and reverses any malabsorption that may have resulted from damage to the cells of your small intestine. With no more malabsorption, the gas and bloating associated with your untreated celiac disease should improve as well.

It's not uncommon, however, for people with celiac disease to have other digestive problems that contribute to bloating even after they get the disease to quiet down on a gluten-free diet. So if you find that some of your bloating symptoms persist even after going strictly gluten-free—and having clean, antibody-free blood tests to prove it—you should explore the other sections of this book to help identify other possible causes. Common ones include SIBO (chapter 8), which people can develop during the active inflammatory phase of their untreated celiac disease; constipation (chapter 7), which can worsen for some people on a gluten-free diet when they're eating fewer soluble-fiber rich grains; classic indigestion (chapter 4), which can flare up if you find yourself eating a lot more salads to replace sandwiches on your gluten-free diet; or carbohydrate intolerances (chapter 9), which can surface in response to fermentable flours and fibers—like inulin and bean flours—used in gluten-free processed foods.

Learn How to Read Labels

To be successful on the gluten-free diet, you're going to need to learn how to read a food label. Unfortunately, it's not enough to just seek out the claim "gluten-free," as current labeling laws allow products that contain ingredients likely to be cross-contaminated with gluten, like conventionally processed oats, to carry a "gluten-free" claim. On the flip side, plenty of foods are naturally gluten-free but aren't necessarily labeled as such; you don't want to limit yourself unnecessarily by skipping over them in favor of foods that carry the GF label. And while it's rare, occasionally a product will be labeled gluten-free despite the label listing that it contains a gluten ingredient! Mistakes can happen, so it's up to you to be vigilant to keep the gluten out of your diet.

If you are a regular label reader, you may have noticed that packaged food products all contain allergen declarations by law; if a food contains wheat, the label explicitly needs to state "CONTAINS: WHEAT" right after the ingredient list. Alas, this is also not a shortcut to avoid label-reading, as products labeled "wheat-free" are not necessarily gluten-free! A food that doesn't contain any wheat may still contain gluten from barley, rye, or ingredients derived from them.

When reading an ingredient list, you'll need to know the many nicknames, alter egos, and pseudonyms that gluten goes by. The alphabetized list below is a pretty good place to start:

Barley	Gluten	Rye
Barley malt	Graham flour	Seitan
Bran	Hydrolyzed vegetable protein (HVP)	Semolina
Bread crumbs		Soy sauce (unless *gluten-free tamari soy sauce* specified)
Bromated flour	Kamut	
Bulgur	Malt (and malt extract, malt flavoring, malt syrup)	Spelt
Cake meal		
Couscous	Matzo meal	Triticale
Durum	Oats, oat flour (unless *gluten-free oats* specified)	Unbromated flour
Einkorn		Wheat
Emmer		Wheat flour, whole-wheat flour
Enriched flour	Orzo	
Farina	Passover cake flour	Wheat starch
Farro	Pastry flour	Wheat germ
Flour	Pearled barley	Wheat bran
	Phyllo (Filo) dough	White flour

Know What Foods Gluten Lives In

If you ever plan to eat comfortably again, you'll have to familiarize yourself with which types of foods gluten is commonly found in. Since the word *gluten* does not appear in flashing lights on every packaged food or restaurant menu item that contains it, it may be helpful to consult

Wheat	Bread, toast, rolls, wraps, flour tortillas (burritos, fajitas, and quesadillas), bagels, pita, english muffins, croissants, pizza crusts
	Pasta, macaroni, gnocchi, orzo, udon, soba noodles, lo mein noodles, Chinese-style noodles, ramen noodles
	Wontons, dumplings, pierogis, gyoza, ravioli
	Couscous
	Pancakes, waffles, french toast, crepes
	Flour, bread crumbs, panko, matzo meal (and foods made from them, like breaded chicken cutlets, battered/fried foods)
	Crackers, breadsticks, pita chips, pretzels, matzo
	Farina, Cream of Wheat, Wheatena
	Many cold cereals, including bran cereals
	Cookies, cakes, muffins, pastries, scones (including corn bread and corn muffins)
	Many energy bars, protein bars, fiber bars, and granola bars
	Gravies, thick sauces (especially white, yellow, or brown colored)
	Asian dishes, marinades, or dressings prepared with soy sauce
	Beer and ingredients derived from it (e.g., brewer's yeast)
	Communion wafers
Barley	Barley-containing soups or stews
	Some multigrain breakfast cereals
	Barley malt flavoring (potato chips, crisped rice cereals, other snack foods)
	Beer
	Malt vinegar
	Malt liquor-based drinks
	Coffee substitutes (e.g., Pero)
Rye	Rye bread
	Certain Scandinavian-style crispbread crackers (e.g., Wasa, Ryvita, Finn Crisp)
	Pumpernickel bread or crackers
	Cold or hot multigrain cereals

these reference lists regularly as you're adapting to the GF diet—particularly when planning to dine out at a new type of restaurant.

Watch Out for Hidden Gluten

The fundamentals of a gluten-free diet are pretty straightforward, and it doesn't take long to master the art of reading a food label to determine whether a food is safe for you to eat or not. It's much harder for newcomers to the gluten-free diet to anticipate all the places gluten can hide on a restaurant menu, in the medicine cabinet, at your local café, in holiday foods, in religious ceremonies, and in your kids' Halloween candy pail.

TABLE 10.1: **Where Gluten Hides**

Restaurants	
	JAPANESE
	Soy sauce (and any dish made with it as a marinade)
	Ginger dressing served on salads
	Miso soup (miso paste may be barley based)
	Imitation crab (used in California rolls), also known as surimi
	"Crunch" topping on sushi rolls, like on volcano rolls
	Tempura
	Udon, ramen, or soba noodles
	Teriyaki-glazed fish or meats
	CONTINENTAL
	All sandwiches served on bread, buns, rolls, and wraps
	Meatballs, meat loaf, veggie burgers, some turkey or salmon burgers, crab cakes, and any other protein food that needs a "binder" (often bread crumbs)
	Gravies and any white-, yellow-, or brown-colored sauce (they use flour)
	Fried foods that are breaded/battered, like mozzarella sticks, crispy shrimp
	Fried foods that may share the same deep fryer with breaded/battered foods (including french fries)
	Pan-seared chicken or fish (it's likely flour-dusted)
	Soups or mashed potatoes made from a mix
	STEAK HOUSE
	Battered/fried appetizers (e.g., onion rings, breaded shrimp)
	Crab cakes
	Crouton-containing salads or breaded goat cheese atop salads
	Mac and cheese side
	Most desserts
	ITALIAN
	Pasta and pizza dishes
	Breaded/battered appetizers (fried calamari)
	Stuffed mushrooms/veggies (often contain bread crumbs)
	Salads with croutons
	Chicken/eggplant Parmesan (cutlets are breaded)
	Chicken or meat dishes served in a non-tomato-based sauce, like marsala sauce (sauce often thickened with flour)
	CHINESE
	Lo mein or other noodle dishes
	Wontons, dumplings
	Egg rolls
	Most brown sauces/condiments used for stir-fries (they'll contain soy sauce and/or oyster sauce, which contain gluten)
	Pancakes served with Mu Shu dishes
	Battered/fried meat dishes

MEXICAN

Burritos

Fajitas and quesadillas (though you can ask that they be prepared with corn tortillas instead of flour)

SOUTHEAST ASIAN (THAI, VIETNAMESE)

Stir-fries made with soy sauce, dark soy sauce, or oyster sauce (ask)

Noodle dishes made with egg noodles or wheat noodles instead of rice noodles

Fried appetizers like spring rolls, fried wontons

Curry puffs

Crispy shallots (topping used in Vietnamese soups)

Bánh mì (Vietnamese sandwiches, served on bread)

SOUTH ASIAN/WEST INDIAN

Breads: naan, paratha, poori, chapati, roti

Appetizers: samosas, sometimes vegetable pakoras

Farina-based dishes

Dosas (large Southern Indian crepes): the batter and/or certain fillings (farina)

Desserts: gulab jamun, pastries

Medicine Cabinet	Pills whose coatings or fillers are made with wheat starch
	Fiber supplements made with wheat dextrin
	Modified food starch or *starch* listed as an inactive ingredient
Candy Jar	Licorice (including Twizzlers)
	Jordan almonds
	Chocolate-coated crisped rice pieces, wafers, or cookies
	Malt balls (e.g., Whoppers)
Holidays and Religious	Communion wafers (gluten-free available)
	Passover matzo (gluten-free available)
	Note: A "Kosher for Passover" label does not denote gluten-free
Café Beverages	Certain pumpkin-spiced coffee drinks
	Lattes flavored with certain brands/flavors of syrups that are not gluten-free
	Herbal teas that contain barley malt as an ingredient (read labels!)
	Coffee substitutes made from barley (e.g., Pero)

Be Aware of Situations Where Cross-Contamination
with Gluten Is Likely

Some people with celiac disease can be triggered by ingesting the amount of gluten present in a bread crumb or two. For this reason, it's not enough to simply avoid eating gluten-containing foods. You also need to watch out for otherwise-safe foods that may have come into enough contact with a gluten-containing food where trace amounts of the gluten wind up on it. Common scenarios where gluten-containing foods and GF foods may comingle include:

- Oatmeal, granolas, and granola bars made from regular oats (that were not processed to keep grains of wheat away). Note: These can carry a gluten-free label claim by law!

- Pizzerias that offer both regular and GF pizza (but may not protect the GF pizza from floured shared surfaces)

- Restaurants that offer both regular and GF pasta (but may not cook them in different water)

- Restaurant french fries (that may share the deep fryer with battered or breaded appetizers like mozzarella sticks, onion rings, breaded shrimp, etc.)

- Shared pop-up toaster ovens used for regular bread and GF bread (where crumbs can intermingle)

- Shared jars of peanut butter, cream cheese, jelly, or butter in homes with both regular and GF bread (double-dipping can transfer crumbs into jar)

This chapter marks the end of the section on bloating that originates in the intestines. If you didn't recognize your brand of bloating in this malabsorption chapter, then I recommend you revisit your quiz results to see whether there's another chapter description that better fits how you feel. But if you feel confident that you've isolated a probable cause of your bloating, then let's move on to part 4 and dive deeper into strategies for using fiber to your advantage and the therapeutic diet most likely to help you manage your bloating once and for all!

PART IV

DIETARY REMEDIES
FOR BLOATING

11.

Flexing Fiber
to Your Advantage

FIBER MAY BE THE MOST misunderstood nutrient out there. Most of my patients arrive with a pretty one-dimensional view of it, believing that fiber's only attributes are helping people go to the bathroom and making people gassy. The reality, however, is so much more complex! When you are plagued with bloating, understanding the nuances of different types of fiber can be a secret weapon that helps you eat the healthiest possible diet while achieving the best symptom control.

What Is Fiber, and Why Should I Eat It?

Fiber is a group of carbohydrates that comes from plants. Fiber differs from other types of plant carbohydrates by virtue of the fact that human beings lack the digestive enzymes to break it down and extract energy from it. This has two implications:

- First, fiber is, by definition, indigestible. It *will* show up in your poop, and brightly colored forms of high-fiber foods will be especially visible. Corn kernels, tomato or pepper skins, kiwi seeds, flaxseeds, blueberry skins, wrinkled spinach leaves, nut pieces, quinoa threads . . . if you see these in your stool, don't be alarmed! It doesn't mean you don't tolerate these foods, and it doesn't mean you didn't absorb the nutrients from these foods, either. It just means that the fiber is doing its job. You'll likely see more fiber in a less-formed, looser stool than you see in a more-formed stool, because more of the stool contents are exposed.

- Second, fiber provides a very minimal number of calories. When a food is indigestible by digestive enzymes in the small intestine, it means that its stored energy (calories) cannot be accessed. (Although very modest numbers of calories may be liberated when your gut's bacteria ferment certain types of fibers once they reach the colon.) Since fiber takes up space in the stomach but doesn't provide much by way of calories, eating a higher-fiber diet often helps you control your weight. It fills you up and crowds out portions of more calorie-dense foods.

To be clear: Since fiber, by definition, comes from plants, all animal-derived proteins (eggs, meat, chicken, fish, cheese) do not contain any fiber, nor do any pure fats like oils or butter. Plant-based proteins like beans, nuts, and seeds, however, *do* contain fiber in addition to other digestible nutrients like protein, fat, and/or some digestible starches.

There are many, many health benefits associated with eating a diet rich in fiber from a variety of foods. People who eat high-fiber diets are less likely to become overweight or to develop type 2 diabetes or heart disease. People who already have type 2 diabetes are better able to manage their blood sugars on a high-fiber diet, and people who already have heart disease are better able to manage their cholesterol levels on a high-fiber diet. High-fiber diets are protective against a variety of different cancers, especially cancers of the digestive system: colon cancer, esophageal cancer, and stomach cancer. In other words, there are many compelling health reasons to eat the highest-fiber diet you can comfortably tolerate.

Patients often ask me how much fiber they should eat in a day. It's a difficult question to answer, because everyone's body is different in terms of its fiber needs and tolerance. From a purely objective health standpoint, it's recommended that women eat 25 grams of fiber per day, and men should aim for 38 grams per day. (For context, the average American typically gets somewhere around 11–14 grams per day.) If you're interested in tracking your fiber intake to see how your typical diet compares, you can adjust the settings on most electronic food journal apps—like MyFitnessPal or FatSecret—to track your fiber automatically when you log your food.

But when you've got digestive issues, there's no textbook formula for the "right" amount of fiber. I've had chronically constipated female patients who can barely eke out a bowel movement every three days on a diet with over 40 grams of fiber daily, plus the maximum dose of magnesium supplements. And on the other end of the spectrum, I've had patients severely bloated from gastroparesis who can poop reasonably regularly even though they barely tolerate ten grams of fiber per day from soft and puréed forms like fruit smoothies and puréed veggie soups. The right amount of fiber for you is the highest amount that you can comfortably tolerate and that helps you manage your digestive symptoms.

The Different Attributes of Fiber

All fiber is not the same. There are different types of fiber in our food supply, and these behave very differently inside our digestive tracts. They differ on a few key dimensions:

- **Moisture-Holding Potential:** A key difference in fiber types relates to their moisture-holding potential, or how well they can dissolve in water. Soluble fiber dissolves in water, forming a viscous, gel-like texture that helps hold on to moisture in your stool, keeping it soft, formed, and easy to pass. Think of soluble fiber as "poo glue" that holds all the little pieces together into a more complete log that can be easily passed in one fell swoop. Insoluble fiber cannot dissolve in water, which means its effect on stool texture is to make it bulky but not necessarily cohesive. If you need a mental image, picture what happens when you pour a packet of instant oatmeal into water: It absorbs it like a sponge, getting thick and gummy in the process. That's what soluble fiber does in your gut. Now picture what happens if you dip a big piece of lettuce into water: It simply becomes a wet piece of lettuce without changing its form at all. That's what happens to insoluble fiber in your gut—it remains intact and contributes to more substantial, bulkier stools but generally can't hold on to moisture very well.

A diet predominant in insoluble fiber may result in your having more little pieces of poop rather than longer, intact logs. If your colon's transit time is normal, these pieces may be soft, fluffy, or "shredded wheaty" in appearance. If your colon's transit time is slow, these pieces may be hard little balls that resemble rabbit pellets. For constipated people, a balance of both types of fiber is generally ideal—some insoluble fiber whose bulkiness will stimulate the sluggish colon to keep chugging along, and some soluble fiber to help keep the stool moist, formed, and easy to pass when it finally arrives at the finish line.

- Effect on the Transit Time in Your Digestive Tract: Largely as the result of its bulkiness and inability to hold on to moisture, insoluble fiber speeds up the transit time of food and waste moving through the gut, making it especially helpful for people with slow-transit constipation. In contrast, soluble fiber's thick, gooey, viscous properties slow down transit time in the gut, making it especially helpful for people who suffer from diarrhea, too-frequent bowel movements, or too-urgent bowel movements. It can absorb some of that extra water that would otherwise make stools too loose, improve the form of your stools, and consolidate those multiple trips to the bathroom by allowing you to pass more of your stool in a single go.

- Fermentability (Gassiness Potential): Some types of fiber, nicknamed *high FODMAP,* are easily fermented by the bacteria in your colon, making them more likely to provoke lots of gas. Other types of fiber, nicknamed *low FODMAP,* are not easily fermented by the bacteria in your colon, making them less likely to provoke lots of gas. Chapter 13 has lots more detail about FODMAPs, but for now, just remember that high FODMAP is shorthand for "potentially gassier" and low FODMAP is shorthand for "less likely to be gassy."

What Are the Best Types of Fiber for Me?

People who don't have any digestive complaints need not give much thought to the types, textures, and amounts of fiber they consume, but if you're reading this book, chances are you *do* need to give these issues some thought. For this reason, I find it helpful to group the different fiber-rich foods into categories based on whether they're more soluble or insoluble and whether they're more fermentable or less fermentable. With this classification, you can identify those fiber-rich foods most likely to agree with you digestively.

While individual tolerances vary, there are two rules of thumb when it comes to fiber choice and bloating:

- When you're prone to any kind of bloating, the most universally tolerated plant foods are soluble-fiber rich and low FODMAP.
  These are the fiber-rich foods least stimulating to the digestive tract in terms of stomach stretch, colon motility, and gassiness potential. See the lower-left quadrant of table 7.1 below for examples of foods that meet these criteria.

- When you're prone to any kind of bloating, the least universally tolerated plant foods are insoluble-fiber rich and high FODMAP.
  While those whose bloating originates in the stomach can often get away with eating foods in this category as long as its texture has been tamed into a soup, smoothie, or spread, the fact remains that consuming these foods in their whole, unmodified form will be problematic for people with a variety of different bloating types. See the upper-right quadrant of table 11.1 for examples of foods that meet these criteria.

As far as the foods that fall into the other categories, your tolerance will likely depend more on your type of bloating.

TABLE 11.1: Properties of Common Fiber-Rich Foods

	Soluble-Fiber Rich	Insoluble-Fiber Rich
Higher FODMAP	(Skinless) apples, applesauce	Artichokes
	Apricots	Beans (black, white, pinto)
	Avocados	Blackberries
	Beets	Cabbage
	Broccoli florets	Celery
	Cauliflower florets	Cherries
	Jicama	Chickpeas/garbanzo beans
	Mangoes	Edamame (boiled soybeans)
	Mushrooms	Kale
	Nectarines	Lentils
	Onions	Peas
	Peaches	Pomegranate seeds
	Pears	Wheat bran
	Pearled barley	
	Plums/prunes	
	Watermelon	
Lower FODMAP	Cantaloupe	Arugula
	Carrots	Bean sprouts
	Chia seeds	Blueberries
	Clementines	Bok choy
	(Peeled) cucumbers	Corn on the cob/kernels
	Green beans (string beans)	Fennel
	Honeydew	Flaxseeds (2 teaspoons max)
	Kiwis	Grapes
	Oatmeal, oat bran, oat flour	Lettuce (all varieties)
	Oranges	Peanuts
	Papayas	Peppers
	Quinoa	Pineapples
	(Skinless) sweet potato	Popcorn
	Tangerines	Pumpkin seeds (pepitas)
	Winter squash (acorn, kabocha, pumpkin)	Sesame seeds
	Yellow squash	Spinach
	Zucchini	Strawberries
		Sunflower seeds

If Your Bloating Originates in the Stomach

Whether from gastroparesis (GP), abdomino-phrenic dyssynergia (APD), indigestion, or functional dyspepsia (FD), the texture and form of the fiber-rich foods you choose may matter more than whether their fiber is soluble or insoluble, high FODMAP or low FODMAP. Because insoluble fiber–rich foods tend to be very bulky and tough in texture—think roughage like leafy greens, fruit and vegetable skins, seeds, and bran—these foods in an unmodified form commonly provoke bloating unless they've been juiced, peeled and cooked, puréed into soups, or ground into a fine flour. A kale salad with sliced apples would be a nightmare, but a small kale smoothie with an apple juice base should be fine.

Foods with more soluble fiber are likely to be less bloat-inducing even when eaten in a relatively unmodified form, because they're generally softer, moister, and therefore faster to empty the stomach. Soluble fiber–rich foods are cooked grains and the inside flesh of (peeled, seedless) fruits or root vegetables like beets and carrots. Chapter 12 offers examples of how to enjoy foods from both categories in a texture-appropriate way. The FODMAP content of a food should not matter much if your bloating originates in the stomach—unless you're also prone to constipation and farting from issues that originate in the intestines. FODMAPs don't provoke gas in the stomach, as there are no bacteria living there. Therefore, texture-appropriate forms of even higher-FODMAP foods like bean spreads and puréed cauliflower soups may work perfectly well for you.

If your bloating results from an intolerance to a certain type of higher-FODMAP carbohydrate found in beans or certain vegetables, then you'll be most comfortable with the lower-FODMAP fiber sources in general; these are found in table 11.1. Chapter 13 offers lengthier lists of which foods contain which higher-FODMAP carbohydrates beyond sugars so you can build on the basic list of safe fiber-rich foods above with additional options tailored to your particular intolerance.

If Your Bloating Originates in the Intestines

You'll need to be more careful about the FODMAPiness of your fiber sources, because higher-FODMAP foods will contribute to more intestinal gas. High-FODMAP sources of fiber are almost universally problematic for those with SIBO, and they can also be quite uncomfortable for people with constipation who are very backed up with stool. But all low-FODMAP sources of fiber—whether they're predominantly soluble or insoluble—are usually well tolerated by most people with SIBO until it's treated successfully.

If you're constipated and FOS, the gas generated from high-FODMAP foods can get trapped behind bottlenecked stool and cause lots of gas pain and bloating. (Once you get things moving along better and can reduce the stool backlog, you may be able to tolerate higher-FODMAP sources of fiber more comfortably.) If your constipation is caused by irritable bowel syndrome (IBS) or slow colonic transit time, then all types of low-FODMAP fiber may be tolerated well—both soluble fiber predominant and insoluble. If your constipation is caused by pelvic floor dysfunction, you'll want to limit how much insoluble fiber you eat and stick to smaller amounts of low-FODMAP, soluble fiber until your condition has been treated effectively. Since your muscles involved in defecation can't pass stool effectively, piling on loads and loads of fiber just adds to the backlog. If much of this fiber is of the insoluble variety, it can get very dried out while waiting around, potentially leading to obstructions (blockages).

If your bloating results from malabsorbing lactose, fructose, or sugar alcohols, both soluble and insoluble fiber types should be tolerated equally well so long as they don't contain the particular sugar you react to! The tables in chapter 9 offer specific foods you'll need to avoid if you are intolerant to fructose or sugar alcohols. Anything not on those lists should be fair game to include in your diet. There is no lactose in any fiber-containing foods.

Fiber Supplements

Fiber supplements are generally used to treat irregular or problematic bathroom patterns when diet change alone doesn't get the job done sufficiently. Soluble-fiber supplements are best used to slow down a speedy gut prone to diarrhea or to help people who are able to move their bowels regularly but feel "incompletely emptied" after going. Insoluble-fiber supplements and psyllium husk supplements (which are a blend of the two fiber types) are best used to speed up a sluggish gut prone to constipation. Examples of all these different types of fiber supplements, including brand names, are described in chapter 14.

But if you are prone to bloating in addition to your bathroom issues, you'll want to be thoughtful when choosing a fiber supplement. Fiber supplements can be very helpful or very aggravating to a bloated belly, depending on your type of bloating and the type of fiber supplement you're considering. Fiber slows down stomach emptying, so people with the types of bloating that originate in the stomach—particularly gastroparesis (GP), abdomino-phrenic dyssynergia (APD), and functional dyspepsia (FD)—typically don't do well with them. Fiber supplements don't often trigger sour stomach bloating, however, so if you're prone to bouts of indigestion but also have troubles in the bathroom, a fiber supplement may be a helpful addition to your regimen.

If you have a type of bloating that originates in the intestines, the tolerability of a fiber supplement will depend on the type of bloating you experience.

- People with constipation from pelvic floor dysfunction should consult a doctor before using a fiber supplement. If your muscles cannot coordinate properly to allow stool to pass, then overloading your system with lots of extra fiber in supplement form may actually make bloating worse, not better. But if the nature of your pelvic floor dysfunction has to do with overly lax muscles or a rectocele (see chapter 7), a soluble-fiber supplement could help bulk up your stools and make them easier for you to pass.

- Some people with IBS or slow-transit constipation may tolerate a fiber supplement, but it's generally not my first recommendation. My patients who are really backed up have described feeling like they've "swallowed a brick" when trying supplemental fiber, as it feels like it just gets stuck behind the stool backlog. My patients with mild opioid-induced constipation (OIC), however, seem to do quite well with fiber supplements in addition to the over-the-counter laxative medications or supplements described in chapters 7 and 14. But in severe cases of OIC, I'd skip the fiber supplements; it can result in stools that are veritable bricks.

- If you have diarrhea from SIBO, a soluble-fiber supplement can sometimes help improve your stool's form and reduce feelings of urgency and frequency of trips to the bathroom without making your bloating any worse. Lower-FODMAP forms of fiber like Citrucel or Benefiber are going to be better tolerated than more fermentable types of fiber marketed as *prebiotic*. See page 290 for examples of these prebiotic fibers. I'd also avoid any fiber supplement that contains probiotics; you've got enough bacteria to contend with without introducing more onto the scene.

- Fiber supplements are unlikely to help if you have bloating or bowel irregularity caused by other types of malabsorption, like lactose intolerance, fructose intolerance, celiac disease, or severe pancreatic insufficiency. If you do have well-controlled celiac disease and would like to use a fiber supplement to address digestive issues unrelated to your celiac—like constipation or diarrhea from irritable bowel syndrome (IBS)—a fiber supplement should be as well tolerated for you as for anyone else. Just make sure to choose a gluten-free brand; see chapter 14 for examples.

12.

The GI Gentle Diet

MODIFYING THE TEXTURE OF YOUR diet can help alleviate bloating or abdominal pain that originates in the stomach, which typically worsens immediately after eating. Softer-textured diets allow the stomach to empty more quickly after eating, which means the stomach won't release acid for too long of a time. Softer-textured meals also minimize the colon-stimulating stretch of the stomach after a meal that can sometimes cause lower-abdominal cramping in people with backed-up bloating (chapter 7).

The GI Gentle diet is composed of moist, soft foods and liquids. It can be high fiber, low fiber, or somewhere in between depending on your needs and tolerances. Most fiber, though, should come from ripe skinless fruit, well-cooked vegetables, and softer-textured grains. These will empty the stomach relatively faster since they lack peels, skins, bran, and coarse-textured chunks whose large particle sizes can take a long time to be broken down. Fiber-containing foods like leafy greens, cabbage slaws, stringier fruits or fruits with lots of skins or seeds, beans, nuts, and seeds should be avoided unless they are very well puréed. Many people following this diet over the long term find that buying a high-powered blender like a Vitamix is worth the investment.

Typically, GI Gentle dieters should go easy on the fat, which means avoiding fried foods; rich sauces like alfredo, carbonara, or cream sauce; and fattier meats like ground lamb, pork or beef ribs, and duck. This is because fat slows down stomach emptying and can prolong the experience of "food baby" type bloating described in chapter 3 or uncomfortable stomach stretch from functional dyspepsia (chapter 5). Since high-fat meals can also trigger acid reflux, they're a nightmare for folks prone to sour stomach bloating (chapter 4).

Fruits

Fruit can always be included in a GI Gentle diet, and eating it regularly should help keep things running smoothly in the bathroom even without lots of roughage in your diet. The trick is to choose fruit with a texture that will liquefy quickly in the stomach so it won't need to spend too much time there waiting for the gastric acid to work its magic.

Portions are an important consideration with fruit when following a GI Gentle diet. For example, watermelon's soft texture is perfect, but when my patients go overboard with portions, they still wind up bloated after eating it. Smoothies pose a similar problem; their liquid texture is perfect for someone on a GI Gentle diet, but it's easy to chug down very large portions of them quickly, causing significant belly bulge. Smoothies sold by retail chains are routinely in the 16-ounce to 32-ounce range; that's one to two quarts of thick liquid that you can guzzle in mere minutes if you're not paying attention. Choose smaller sizes in the 8-ounce to 16-ounce range, and sip them slowly over the course of an hour.

If you also suffer from acid reflux, certain fruits higher in acid may bother you, though they do not necessarily worsen reflux itself. If your reflux is well controlled, these more acidic fruits may not bother you at

Instead of these highly textured fruits . . .	Try these softer-textured alternatives
FRUITS WITH LOTS OF SKINS, THICK SKINS, STRINGY MEMBRANES, OR LOTS OF SEEDS, LIKE: Apples Berries* Cherries Grapefruit and pomelos* Grapes Pineapples* Passion fruit* Persimmons Pomegranate seeds	**SOFT, RIPE, SKINLESS, OR VERY THIN-SKINNED FRUITS WITHOUT SEEDS, LIKE:** Apricots (2 per sitting) Bananas Clementines (2 per sitting) Soft ripe pears (1 per sitting) Soft, ripe melons: cantaloupe, honeydew, and watermelon (up to 2 cups cut melon per sitting) Papayas (1–2 cups per sitting) Soft peaches, plums, and nectarines (1 medium-size fruit per sitting) Ripe mangoes (especially Ataúlfo/champagne/Haitian mangoes); 1 medium-size fruit per sitting Canned pineapples and other canned fruits
DRIED FRUIT WITH TOUGH, LEATHERY TEXTURES, LIKE: Raisins Dates Prunes Dried apricots Dried mangoes Dried figs	**PURÉED FRUITS, LIKE:** Children's squeezable fruit purée pouches Prune juice or pear nectar Fruit smoothies made with some of the fruits in the left column, very well puréed and sipped slowly over the course of an hour Frozen fruit popsicles made with 100% puréed fruit or fruit and yogurt **COOKED FRUITS, LIKE:** Applesauce Baked apples (skinless) Compote made from finely chopped dried fruits Cranberry sauce

all. On the chart above, foods that may not be suited for people with acid reflux—even in a texture-modified form—are indicated with an asterisk (*).

Vegetables

The trick to not gaining too much weight or becoming insanely constipated on a GI Gentle diet is to include texture-friendly vegetables in your diet regularly. Unfortunately, raw vegetables in general and salads in particular are some of the biggest triggers for people whose bloating originates in the stomach. Some people can tolerate small appetizer-size salads comfortably, especially when they're made with softer baby greens instead of tough romaine hearts and iceberg lettuce. If you have sour stomach bloating (chapter 4), small salads will be best tolerated when they're eaten toward the end of the meal rather than at the outset. Still, you'll need to broaden your horizons beyond the "kitchen sink" salad in order to make vegetables work for you. Some recipes are included toward the end of this chapter.

Certain vegetables are high in naturally occurring nitrites that can cause reflux in susceptible people, particularly when raw or juiced. Some high-acid vegetables like tomatoes can aggravate symptoms of acid reflux in susceptible people. On the chart below, such higher-acid or higher-nitrite vegetables are indicated with an asterisk (*). Because these are super-nutritious foods, I only recommend avoiding them if they actually provoke reflux symptoms for you personally.

Instead of these highly textured vegetables . . .	Try these softer-textured alternatives
RAW SALADS, ESPECIALLY ENTRÉE-SIZE: Iceberg lettuce Romaine lettuce Raw spinach Raw kale **CABBAGE, INCLUDING:** Slaw/coleslaw Sauerkraut	Roasted beet and goat cheese salad Avocado salad with minimal raw greens Asian-style pickled cucumber salad* made with peeled and seeded cucumbers Green juices, tomato juice,* or other vegetable juices (raw beet* or celery* juices may provoke reflux due to their high nitrite content) Gazpacho* Appetizer-size baby greens salad if tolerated (chew very well!)
RAW CRUDITÉ VEGETABLES (E.G., FOR DIPPING IN HUMMUS OR OTHER DRESSINGS OR DIPS), LIKE: Celery sticks* Raw baby carrots Raw pepper slices Raw broccoli or cauliflower florets	**STEAMED, BLANCHED, OR BOILED VEGETABLES FOR DIPPING; LIMIT TO 1 CUP SERVING PER SITTING:** Steamed baby carrots Well-steamed broccoli or cauliflower florets Roasted, peeled red peppers from a jar

COOKED VEGETABLES THAT RETAIN THEIR THICK, WOODY, FIBROUS, OR STRINGY TEXTURES, SUCH AS:	SOFTER, COOKED VEGETABLES (AIM FOR ½ CUP TO 1 CUP SERVING PER SITTING):
Sautéed broccoli rabe/rapini	Chopped, steamed, or boiled spinach*
Cooked kale and collard greens	Boiled green beans
Steamed, roasted, or sautéed asparagus stalks	Cooked winter squash (acorn, butternut, kabocha) and pumpkin
Roasted parsnips	Cooked carrots
Sugar snap peas or snow peas	Cooked summer squash (zucchini and yellow squash; preferably without seeds)
Steamed artichokes	Spiralized vegetable noodles ("zoodles")
Cooked eggplant (with skins and seeds)	Cooked eggplant without skins
Brussels sprouts	Cooked asparagus tips
Cabbage	Roasted or boiled beets*
	Well-steamed/roasted cauliflower florets, cauliflower "rice," or mashed cauliflower
	Well-steamed / boiled broccoli florets
	Jarred artichoke hearts
	Well-sautéed peppers, mushrooms, and onions*
	Vegetable soups (aim for 12–16-ounce serving per sitting)

Grains

On a GI Gentle diet, you'll likely do best with some combination of refined grains and somewhat processed whole-grain foods where the particle size of the fiber has been ground pretty finely into flour—think tender whole-grain sandwich breads, crackers, flake cereals, and frozen waffles. For example, consider the texture difference between cooked steel-cut oats and Cheerios, which are both made from whole oats. While both are whole-grain foods, the chewy texture and intact bran of the steel-cut oats will take far longer to empty from the stomach than the finely milled whole-oat flour used to make Cheerios.

You'll also want to consider the relative amount of fiber in certain whole grains compared to others. Although both are whole grains, brown rice has far less fiber than barley. Therefore, it is more likely to sit well in the bellies of people whose bloating originates in the stomach.

Experimenting with both whole grains and refined grains will help you land on the healthiest diet you can comfortably tolerate. So will paying attention to the physical properties of the food itself; think about how the texture looks and feels when a food is cooked and well chewed. If a toddler could swallow it easily, you're on the right track.

Instead of these highly textured grain-based foods ...	Try these softer-textured alternatives
HIGH-FIBER (>5 GRAMS PER SERVING) BREAKFAST CEREALS, INCLUDING:	**REFINED-TEXTURE, MODERATE FIBER (3–4 GRAMS PER SERVING) CEREALS THAT CONTAIN SOME WHOLE GRAINS, INCLUDING:**
Shredded wheat–type cereals, including Weetabix and Mini Wheats	Wheaties, Total, Oat Bran Flakes, Cheerios, Life, Barbara's Puffins, or Multigrain Spoonfuls
Bran flakes, including Raisin Bran	Cascadian Farms Multigrain Squares
Grape Nuts	**LOW-FIBER CEREALS (1–2 GRAMS PER SERVING), INCLUDING:**
High-fiber "twig" cereals like All Bran, Bran Buds, Fiber One, Kashi Go Lean, and Trader Joe's Twigs, Flakes & Clusters	Special K, Rice Krispies, Kix, Corn Flakes, Chex varieties (except Wheat Chex), Crispix
Granola and muesli	*Note: The low-fiber cereals listed above can provoke high blood sugar levels in people with normal stomach-emptying time due to their easy digestibility. As such, they may not be an ideal choice for people with pre-diabetes or type 2 diabetes.*
DENSELY TEXTURED, CHEWY, COOKED WHOLE GRAINS, SUCH AS:	**LOWER-FIBER OR LESS-TEXTURED COOKED WHOLE GRAINS AND REFINED GRAINS (UP TO 1 CUP PER SITTING):**
Steel-cut oatmeal or rolled oats	Quick-cooking oats or instant oatmeal
Barley	Farina, cream of rice, or cream of buckwheat cooked cereals
Wheat berries	Couscous (regular or whole wheat)
Wild rice	Brown rice
Millet	White rice (includes yellow rice)
Sorghum	Polenta or grits
Whole-wheat pasta	Quinoa
HIGH-FAT NOODLE DISHES, SUCH AS:	Regular pasta, macaroni, and noodles
	Soba noodles
Instant ramen noodles	Rice noodles
Take-out lo mein noodles	Skinless baked potato or baked sweet potato
Heavily seeded or thick-crusted "rustic" bakery breads	Soft whole-wheat sandwich bread with 2 grams or less of fiber per slice (limit 2 slices per sitting)
Dense, dark European brick-style whole-grain and seed breads (e.g., Mestemacher)	**REFINED-GRAIN BREADS, INCLUDING:**
	White (sandwich bread, English muffins)
	Sourdough
	Rye
	Bagels (If large New York–style, limit to ½ bagel per sitting)

Heavily seeded crackers or highly textured "woven whole wheat" crackers (e.g., Triscuits)	WHOLE-GRAIN CRACKERS MADE FROM MILLED WHOLE-GRAIN FLOUR WITH UP TO 3 GRAMS FIBER PER SERVING, SUCH AS:
Dense, rustic, Scandinavian-style crispbreads like original Wasa, Finn Crisp, or GG Bran Crispbreads	Wheat Thins
	Kashi Fire Roasted Veggie crackers
	Wasa Crisp & Light crispbreads
	Brown Rice Cakes (gluten-free)
	Le Pain des Fleurs Crispbreads (gluten-free)
	REFINED-GRAIN CRACKERS AND CHIPS, SUCH AS:
	Pita chips
	"Popped corn" chips or popcorn-style rice cakes
	Pretzels
	Soda crackers, water crackers, rice crackers, buttery rounds, cheese crackers, saltines
	Nut Thins

Proteins and Dairy Foods

Protein foods, especially animal protein foods, are naturally free of fiber, making them easy for the stomach to liquefy and empty. For this reason, people with various forms of stomach bloating typically tolerate them well. The notable exceptions are very high-fat meats and gooey, cheesy entrées, which can take quite a long time to empty the stomach due to their high fat content. Ditto for leaner proteins like chicken, fish, and shrimp that are battered and fried. High-fat foods are also likely to provoke acid reflux in susceptible people and are therefore best avoided, particularly among those with gastroparesis (chapter 3) and sour stomach bloating (chapter 4).

Plant-based protein foods like nuts, seeds, and beans do contain fiber, however. Therefore, you'll need to pay attention to their texture and portion to ensure they'll clear the stomach quickly and without too much bloat-inducing stretch. For all foods in general and these foods in particular, taking time to chew very well is essential!

A final thing to consider about beans in particular is their well-deserved reputation for generating intestinal gas (farts) even when they're in a smooth, puréed texture like hummus. If this isn't a problem for you, then look for the texture-friendly beans in the table below and go for it! If you already suffer from problematic levels of intestinal gas, though, it's best to skip beans or use an alpha-galactosidase enzyme supplement to improve their digestibility; see chapters 9 and 14 for more details.

Instead of these slow-digesting protein and dairy foods . . .	Try these alternatives
HIGH-FAT MEATS, SUCH AS: Fatty cuts of steak or tough/chewy cuts (flap steak, porterhouse, skirt steak, New York Strip steak, T-bone, rib eye) Ribs (pork spare ribs, BBQ ribs, beef short ribs, Korean-style Kalbi or Bulgogi) Bacon Lamb (especially ground) Liver **FRIED PROTEIN FOODS, SUCH AS:** Fried chicken Battered/fried Chinese entrées, such as General Tso's chicken, sweet 'n' sour chicken, sesame chicken Fried shrimp and shrimp tempura Fried fish or fish 'n' chips Fatty cold cuts like salami, pastrami, corned beef	**LEAN, MOIST PROTEINS, SUCH AS:** Fish (baked, broiled, steamed, grilled) Lean cold cuts: turkey/turkey pastrami, chicken, ham, roast beef Canadian bacon or turkey bacon Very lean steak (eye of round roast and steak, sirloin tip side steak, top round roast and steak, bottom round roast and steak, top sirloin steak) Eggs, egg whites, egg drop soup Meatballs or meat loaf made from ground turkey, chicken, or veal Tuna salad, chicken salad, egg salad made with low-fat mayonnaise Roasted chicken (e.g., rotisserie) or stewed/braised/baked/grilled chicken thighs Tofu (sautéed, baked, boiled in soup)
LARGE PORTIONS OF FULL-FAT CHEESE, SUCH AS CASSEROLE-TYPE DISHES IN CHEESE SAUCE AND PASTAS WITH CREAM-BASED SAUCES: Homemade macaroni and cheese (most boxed varieties should be fine) Lasagna Cheese fondue Eggplant or chicken Parmesan Deep-dish / cheese-lover pizzas Pasta with alfredo or carbonara sauce Fried mozzarella sticks **CREAM-BASED DESSERTS, SUCH AS:** Premium ice cream (Häagen-Dazs, Ben & Jerry's) Cheesecake Milkshakes Full-fat rice pudding	**CREAMY-TEXTURED, REDUCED-FAT DAIRY PRODUCTS OR DAIRY-FREE ALTERNATIVES** Low-fat cottage cheese Part-skim ricotta Nonfat or low-fat greek yogurt Low-fat regular yogurt or soy yogurt **PORTION CONTROLLED FULL-FAT CHEESE USED AS A SNACK OR GARNISH (LIMIT TO 1 OUNCE PER SITTING)** String cheese or Babybel Sprinkle of feta, goat cheese, or Parmesan on pasta or well-cooked veggies One deli slice of cheese on a lean sandwich (e.g., turkey or ham sandwich) Up to one standard slice of regular pizza in a sitting **LOWER-FAT DAIRY–BASED OR NONDAIRY DESSERTS (LIMIT PORTION TO ½ CUP–1 CUP PER SERVING)** Frozen yogurt Low-fat ice cream Sherbet, sorbet, or frozen fruit popsicles Low-fat pudding or fudgesicles Jell-O

WHOLE BEANS, PEAS, AND LENTILS WITH THEIR SKINS ON LIKE:

Chickpeas

Beans (black, kidney, pinto, white)

Lentils and lentil soups

Split pea soup

Edamame (boiled soybeans)

Peas

WHOLE NUTS OR SEEDS LIKE:

Peanuts, almonds, cashews, pistachios, walnuts, pecans

Pumpkin seeds, sunflower seeds, flax seeds, chia seeds, sesame seeds

KIND bars and other whole nut–based snack bars

PURÉED BEANS AND LENTILS, LIKE:

Hummus

Fat-free refried beans

British-style "smashed peas" (limit ½ cup; see recipe page 192)

SOFT-TEXTURED, BEAN-BASED ENTRÉES LIKE:

Soft-textured veggie burgers (limit one per sitting)

Tofu

Vegetable soups with sparse number of beans (e.g., minestrone)

PURÉED NUTS/SEEDS OR NUT MEAL/ FLOURS, LIKE:

Peanut butter, almond butter, sunflower seed butter (limit 2 tablespoons)

Tahini (limit 2 tablespoons)

Powdered peanut butter (e.g, PB2)

Almond flour

Snack bars made with ground nut butters

A Sample Day on the GI Gentle Diet

Most foods can fit into a soft-textured diet, and it's easy to eat healthily even when salads are off the menu. In fact, the GI Gentle diet can be adapted to any preference. Read on for inspiration!

	Sample Plant-Based Menu	Sample Omnivore Menu	Sample Paleo-Style Menu	Sample Gluten-Free Menu
Breakfast	One packet instant plain oatmeal 1 tablespoon peanut butter mixed in Small banana Cinnamon, maple syrup to taste	2 slices sourdough toast ½ avocado, smashed 2 scrambled egg whites Salt and pepper	3 small chicken or turkey breakfast sausages 1 cup sliced melon or papaya ½ cup coconut milk yogurt	Blend together: 6 ounces low-fat kefir, milk, or almond milk 1 ripe banana 1 cup any frozen fruit (berries, mango, peach, pineapple) 1 scoop whey protein isolate or organic rice protein *or* ⅓ cup pasteurized liquid egg whites
Lunch	1 veggie burger on a slider bun topped with hummus, jarred roasted red pepper, and shavings from one peeled baby cucumber Side of oven-baked sweet potato fries made from ½ medium sweet potato	1–2 sushi rolls (6 pieces each) 1 miso soup	4–6 ounces grilled or baked salmon fillet 1 cup cooked cauliflower rice ½ cup applesauce for dessert	2 soft chicken tacos with a dab of guacamole, refried beans, smooth-textured salsa

continued

	Sample Plant-Based Menu	Sample Omnivore Menu	Sample Paleo-Style Menu	Sample Gluten-Free Menu
Dinner	4 ounces baked tofu ½ cup white rice 1 cup frozen Asian-style stir-fry veggies, steamed and seasoned to taste	½ rotisserie chicken breast (4 ounces) ½ cup mashed potatoes or sweet potatoes 1 cup well-steamed green beans	2 eggs, each baked in ½ of an avocado (15 minutes at 425 degrees) and seasoned with salt, pepper, and/or minced chives ½ cup mashed kabocha squash	4–5 large scallops, pan-seared in butter or olive oil ½ cup polenta or grits ½ cup chopped frozen spinach, sautéed and seasoned to taste
Snack Options	0% greek yogurt or coconut-based nondairy alternative 1 cup smooth carrot-ginger or butternut squash soup 1 ounce dark chocolate 2 small kiwis, peeled	2 clementines or apricots 1 part-skim string cheese ½ cup mango sorbet or frozen fruit pop ⅓ cup guacamole and 1 ounce pita chips	3-ounce can tuna served on 1 ounce baked sweet potato chips Banana with 1 tablespoon almond butter 1 small Paleo-style bar made from soft dried fruit and lean protein like RxBar or Tanka Bar Roasted seaweed sheets	1 rice cake topped with hummus 2 ounces deli-sliced turkey rolled up with 1 ounce reduced-fat swiss cheese ½ cup low-fat pudding (rice, chocolate, tapioca, vanilla) 1 cup watermelon balls

GI Gentle Recipes

While soups, smoothies, omelets, turkey sandwiches, and sushi are easy standbys on the GI Gentle diet, there's no need to get stuck in a rut eating the same old staples. And just because your food needs to be soft, that doesn't mean it needs to be bland. With a little inspiration, you'll find many new favorite dishes that please your palate and keep your bloating at bay.

The recipes that follow are cross-referenced for the low-FODMAP diet (see chapter 13) and contain gluten-free and dairy-free ingredient substitutions so you can home in on those meals best suited for your preferred style of eating. All recipes were developed with sensitivity toward people prone to acid reflux as well; in addition to being low in fat, they're free of garlic and spiciness, use minimal amounts of onion, and are very stingy with acidic ingredients.

BREAKFAST

- Avocado Cilantro Toasts with Scrambled Egg Whites

- Sweet Potato, Sausage, and Kale Frittata

- Mushroom Tofu Scramble
- Get Your Greens Smoothie

SOUPS AND SALADS

- Beet and Goat Cheese Salad with Horseradish Sauce
- Cucumber and Melon Salad
- Asparagus and Rice Soup
- Roasted Butternut Squash and Mushroom Soup

ENTRÉES

- Hawaiian-Style Tuna Poke Bowl
- Salmon Cakes with Mustard-Dill-Yogurt Sauce and Riced Cauliflower
- White Bean and Artichoke Flatbreads
- Turkey, Bell Pepper, and Sweet Potato Hash
- Grilled Fish and Zucchini Tacos with Mango-Avocado Salsa
- Greek-Style Braised Chicken Thighs with Olives and Red Bell Peppers
- Vegetarian Couscous
- Southeast Asian–Flavored Baked Tofu with Shiitake Mushrooms

VEGETABLE SIDE DISHES

- Butternut Squash Spoonbread
- Pub-Style Smashed Peas with Mint
- Roasted Cauliflower "Steaks"
- Moroccan Spiced Carrots

LOW-FAT DESSERTS

- Honey-and-Ginger-Poached Pears
- Peach-Apple Crumble for Two
- Tropical Angel Food Sorbet Cake
- Chocolate-Banana Mousse
- Low-Fat Pumpkin Spice Pillow Cookies

Avocado Cilantro Toasts
with Scrambled Egg Whites 1 SERVING

Crispy toast topped with creamy avocado, softly scrambled egg whites, and crumbled feta cheese makes a light but satisfying breakfast. It is one of my personal favorites because it holds me from breakfast until lunch. I use egg whites rather than whole eggs to offset the fat in the avocado, thereby making it easy to digest. The key to light and fluffy egg whites is not overcooking them.

2 slices fine-crumbed bread of your choice, regular or gluten-free

⅓ large avocado

½ lime

Coarse kosher salt

3 large egg whites or ⅓ cup (generous) liquid egg whites

Olive oil spray or vegetable oil spray

Freshly ground pepper

1 tablespoon crumbled feta cheese

1 tablespoon chopped fresh cilantro

Toast the bread slices and transfer to a plate. Scoop the avocado flesh from its skin and divide between the bread slices. Mash gently with a fork, spreading to cover the toasts. Squeeze a little lime juice over. Sprinkle lightly with salt.

Break or measure the egg whites into a small bowl. Spray a medium non-stick skillet with oil spray, and then place over medium heat and let warm for 30 seconds. Pour the egg whites into the skillet, tipping the pan to spread the whites evenly. Sprinkle lightly with salt and pepper and let stand until the eggs turn white across the bottom, about 1 minute. Using a rubber spatula, scramble the eggs, cooking and stirring just until they turn white throughout and start to firm, about 15 seconds longer. Remove from the heat. Sprinkle the feta and cilantro over the eggs and stir in. Divide the egg whites between the toasts and serve.

Sweet Potato, Sausage, and Kale Frittata

4 SERVINGS

Here's a one-pan meal that is great for breakfast, brunch, lunch, or even weeknight dinners. The recipe features low-fat ingredients, such as nonfat ricotta cheese and a combination of whole eggs and egg whites. Be sure to look for sausage that is lower in fat than most, about 2.5 to 3.5 grams of fat per ounce. A few good choices: Bilinski's, Trader Joe's, Al Fresco, Applegate, and Coleman's.

> 6 large eggs
>
> 4 large egg whites
>
> ½ cup finely grated Parmesan cheese
>
> 2 tablespoons minced fresh basil
>
> ¼ teaspoon coarse kosher salt
>
> Freshly ground pepper
>
> 2 tablespoons extra-virgin olive oil
>
> 2 links chicken-and-apple sausage (see note above), cut lengthwise into quarters, then crosswise into ½-inch pieces
>
> 1 cup coarsely grated peeled sweet potato (about one 4-ounce potato)
>
> 1 cup (packed) baby kale, thinly sliced crosswise
>
> ⅓ cup nonfat ricotta cheese

Preheat the oven to 400°F. Combine the eggs, egg whites, Parmesan cheese, basil, salt, and a little pepper in a medium bowl. Beat with a fork to blend.

Heat 1 tablespoon of the oil in a heavy 10-inch nonstick skillet over medium-high heat. Add the sausage and sauté until beginning to brown, stirring frequently, 1 to 2 minutes. Add the grated sweet potato and cook until it begins to soften, stirring frequently, about 2 minutes. Add the kale and stir just until wilted, about 1 minute. Add the remaining 1 tablespoon oil to the pan and stir to distribute over pan bottom. Add the egg mixture and stir gently to distribute evenly. Reduce the heat to medium. Spoon dollops of ricotta evenly over the eggs. Cook until eggs begin to set on the bottom, about 2 minutes.

Transfer the pan to the oven and bake the frittata until puffed and just set, about 15 minutes. Using a flexible rubber or silicone spatula, free the frittata around the edges. Slide onto a platter or leave in the pan. Serve hot, warm, or at room temperature, cutting into wedges.

NOTE: *To cut the baby kale into thin ribbons (for easy digestion), simply stack the leaves and slice crosswise.*

Mushroom Tofu Scramble 4 SERVINGS

This is perfect for people on a meatless diet and delicious for anyone. I like to serve this nourishing breakfast dish on toast or wrapped in toasted corn tortillas. To make it quickly, prepare the other ingredients while the tofu drains. The secret to including mushrooms in this diet is to cut them into small pieces or slice them thinly, and then cook until very tender.

> 1 14- to 16-ounce package firm tofu
>
> 2 tablespoons extra-virgin olive oil
>
> 2⅔ cups (about 7 ounces) minced mushrooms such as shiitake, crimini, and/or enoki
>
> ¼ onion, minced
>
> Coarse kosher salt
>
> 1 tablespoon soy sauce or tamari
>
> 2 teaspoons minced fresh thyme
>
> Freshly grated Parmesan cheese
>
> Minced green ends of green onions, optional

Drain the tofu, then wrap in 2 layers of paper towels and place on a large plate. Top with another plate and a heavy can. Let drain 15 to 20 minutes. Cut the tofu into about 1-inch pieces, and then crumble with a fork.

Heat the oil in a heavy, large nonstick skillet over medium-high heat. Add the mushrooms and onion. Sprinkle with salt and cook until the mushrooms and onion soften, stirring frequently, about 4 minutes. Add the tofu and stir for 1 minute. Reduce the heat to low, cover, and cook until the vegetables are very tender and flavors blend, stirring occasionally, about 5 minutes. Mix in the soy sauce and thyme. Season to taste with salt.

Divide the scramble among 4 plates. Sprinkle with cheese and green onions, if desired, and serve.

Get Your Greens Smoothie 2 SERVINGS

Indulge in this milkshake-like, nutrient-packed treat for a super-quick breakfast. I enjoy it with only the natural sweetness the berries provide, but you can adjust to taste with a little sugar or maple syrup. If you're on a plant-based diet or simply avoiding dairy, swap out the kefir for a milk substitute of your choice or check out one of the new dairy-free kefirs.

> 1½ cups frozen berries of your choice
> 1 cup plain kefir
> ½ ripe banana, cut into 1-inch pieces
> ½ cup (packed) shredded or chopped kale
> 1 tablespoon hempseed hearts
> ¼ cup nonfat or low-fat milk or milk substitute of your choice
> 1 teaspoon (about) maple syrup or sugar (optional)

Place berries, kefir, banana, kale, and hemp in blender and purée until smooth. Add the milk and blend. Sweeten to taste with syrup or sugar, if desired.

NOTE: *To make this recipe low FODMAP, use lactose-free milk, kefir, almond milk, or coconut milk as your base, substitute spinach for the kale, and limit your berry selection to strawberries, blueberries, or raspberries.*

Beet and Goat Cheese Salad with Horseradish Sauce 4 SERVINGS

Salads are the food that my patients on the GI Gentle diet miss the most, so I've created this one to satisfy that craving. Precooked beets are a cinch to find in the refrigerated section of most supermarkets' produce areas, and they allow this recipe to come together quickly.

12 ounces green beans, trimmed

5 ounces soft fresh goat cheese

1 tablespoon plus 1 teaspoon horseradish

1 tablespoon kefir, nonfat or low-fat milk, or milk substitute of your choice

1½ teaspoons cider vinegar

⅛ teaspoon sugar

1½ tablespoons (about) minced fresh dill

1 8-ounce package steamed and peeled baby beets, drained and sliced into rounds

Cook the green beans in a large pot of boiling salted water until tender, about 12 minutes. Drain well and let cool.

Combine the goat cheese, horseradish, kefir, vinegar, and sugar in a small bowl or mini–food processor. Beat with a handheld beater or process until the sauce is smooth.

Divide the beans among 4 small plates. Drizzle about ½ tablespoon sauce over each serving and sprinkle each generously with dill. Fan the beets over the center of the beans. Drizzle about 1 tablespoon sauce over each. Sprinkle each generously with dill.

NOTE: *The sauce is also great as a dip for cooked green beans.*

Cucumber and Melon Salad 4 SERVINGS

Another salad that is perfect for the GI Gentle diet. This one is super refreshing, so keep it in mind for a hot summer day. Raw cucumbers should work well for most people with sensitive stomachs if they are peeled and shaved into ribbons (avoiding the seeds), and melons are an ideal fruit, since they're soft when ripe and eaten skinless and seedless.

¼ cantaloupe, peeled, then thinly sliced crosswise (about 1½ cups)

¼ mini seedless watermelon, peeled, then thinly sliced crosswise (about 2 cups)

1 small english hothouse cucumber, cut in half crosswise

1 tablespoon fresh lime juice

1 tablespoon extra-virgin olive oil

1 tablespoon chopped fresh mint

1 teaspoon finely grated lime zest

Coarse kosher salt

1 tablespoon crumbled feta cheese

Combine the cantaloupe and watermelon slices in a shallow salad bowl. Remove the peel from the cucumber. Using a vegetable peeler and working around the cucumber, cut the cucumber into thin ribbons, stopping when you reach the seeds.

Add the lime juice, oil, mint, and lime zest to the melons. Sprinkle with salt and toss to coat. Add the cucumber ribbons and feta and toss gently. Taste and add more salt if desired. Divide among 4 plates and serve.

NOTE: *To make this recipe low FODMAP, double the cantaloupe portion and eliminate the watermelon.*

Asparagus and Rice Soup MAKES 4 CUPS

Use this recipe to cook up a pot of comforting soup in about half an hour. Topping with poached eggs transforms it from an appetizer into a filling meal-in-a-bowl. While tarragon is a great match with asparagus, dill and basil are also good choices. The sometimes-woody asparagus stalks are sliced into paper-thin disks for easy digestibility, but the tender tips can be left intact.

12 ounces thin asparagus stalks

2 tablespoons extra-virgin olive oil

½ cup finely chopped onion

4 cups vegetable or chicken broth, plus more if desired

¼ cup white basmati or jasmine rice

1 cup (packed) baby spinach leaves

1 teaspoon fresh lemon juice

1 tablespoon minced fresh tarragon

Coarse kosher salt

Freshly ground pepper

Freshly grated Parmesan cheese

Break off the tough ends of the asparagus where they break naturally and discard. Slice the asparagus stalks into very thin rounds, leaving the tender tips intact.

Heat the oil in a heavy, large saucepan over medium-low heat. Add the onion and sauté until translucent, stirring frequently, about 5 minutes. Add 4 cups of broth and rice and bring to a boil. Reduce the heat, cover, and simmer until the rice is tender, about 15 minutes. Add the sliced asparagus, cover, and simmer until almost tender, about 8 minutes. Add the asparagus tips, cover, and simmer until tender, about 5 minutes. Add the spinach and lemon juice and simmer until spinach is just wilted, about 1 minute. Mix in the tarragon. Season lightly with salt and pepper, and thin with more broth if desired.

Ladle the soup into bowls. Sprinkle each with a little Parmesan cheese and serve.

Roasted Butternut Squash and Mushroom Soup 4 SERVINGS

A velvety purée boasting the flavors of fall, this is lovely before a meal or as a midafternoon snack. Or serve with toast for a satisfying lunch.

> Olive oil spray
>
> 2½-pound butternut squash
>
> 1 tablespoon extra-virgin olive oil, plus more as needed
>
> Coarse kosher salt
>
> Freshly ground pepper
>
> 3 cups chicken broth or vegetable broth, plus more if desired
>
> 8 ounces crimini or button mushrooms, thinly sliced
>
> ¼ onion, minced
>
> 2 teaspoons minced fresh thyme or marjoram
>
> 1 teaspoon ground cumin
>
> 1 tablespoon plus 1 teaspoon sugar (preferably brown)
>
> Freshly grated Parmesan cheese

Preheat the oven to 425°F. Spray a rimmed baking pan with olive oil spray. Cut the squash in half lengthwise and scoop out the seeds and fibers. Brush the cut sides with oil and sprinkle with salt and pepper. Arrange squash halves cut side down on the prepared baking pan. Roast until the squash is tender in the thickest parts, about 1 hour. Cool slightly.

Scrape the squash flesh from the skin and transfer to a food processor (there will be about 2 cups squash flesh). Add ½ cup of the broth and purée until very smooth.

Heat 1 tablespoon oil in a heavy, large saucepan over medium heat. Add the mushroom slices, onion, and 1 teaspoon of the thyme. Sauté until the onion and mushrooms are tender, stirring occasionally, about 8 minutes. Add the cumin and stir until fragrant, about 30 seconds. Add 2½ cups broth. Increase the heat and bring to a boil, stirring up any browned bits. Add the squash purée and bring to a boil. Reduce the heat, cover, and simmer 20 minutes to blend the flavors. Mix in the sugar. Season the soup to taste with salt and a little pepper. Thin to desired consistency with additional broth if desired.

Ladle the soup into bowls. Sprinkle the top of each with about ¼ teaspoon thyme and a little Parmesan cheese.

NOTE: *Roasting fresh squash adds depth of flavor, but to save time, the roasted squash can be replaced with a 15-ounce can of pumpkin or butternut squash. There is no need to purée the canned product with broth; instead, add 3 cups of broth to the pot after sautéing the mushrooms, bring to a boil, and then mix in the canned pumpkin before continuing with the recipe.*

Hawaiian-Style Tuna Poke Bowl 4 SERVINGS

Poke bowls are hugely popular in New York City where I practice and are a convenient alternative to take-out salads for lunch. This version delivers a variety of flavors and textures, qualities that are often lacking on the GI Gentle diet: crunch from paper-thin slices of quick-pickled cucumber and radish, soft-textured blanched carrots and spinach, and tender ahi tuna.

MARINATED CUCUMBER AND RADISHES

1 tablespoon rice wine vinegar

¾ teaspoon sugar

Coarse kosher salt

¼ hothouse cucumber, peeled, halved lengthwise, seeds removed with a spoon, thinly sliced (about ⅓ cup)

3 large radishes, thinly sliced (about ¼ cup)

1 cup white basmati or jasmine rice, rinsed

TUNA AND VEGETABLES

¼ cup soy sauce or tamari

1 tablespoon plus 1 teaspoon minced peeled fresh ginger

2 teaspoons rice wine vinegar

2 teaspoons Asian (toasted) sesame oil

¼ teaspoon (generous) sugar

1 6-ounce bag baby spinach

2 medium carrots, thinly sliced (about 1 cup)

1 pound ahi tuna, cut into ½-inch cubes

2 tablespoons minced green onion tops (green part only)

1 avocado, halved, pit removed

Toasted sesame seeds

FOR THE CUCUMBER AND RADISHES: Combine the vinegar, sugar, and salt in a small bowl. Add 1 tablespoon water and stir to dissolve the sugar and salt. Add the cucumber and radishes. Marinate for at least 10 minutes and up to 1 hour.

Rinse the rice, and place in a small saucepan. Add 1½ cups water. Bring to a boil, reduce the heat to low, cover, and cook until the water is absorbed, 15 to 20 minutes. Turn off the heat and let stand covered 5 minutes. Fluff with a fork, then cover to keep warm.

MEANWHILE, PREPARE THE TUNA AND VEGETABLES: Combine the soy sauce, ginger, vinegar, sesame oil, and sugar in a medium bowl and stir the soy-ginger sauce to blend.

Bring a large saucepan of salted water to a boil. Add the spinach and cook just until wilted, 10 to 20 seconds. Using a slotted spoon, transfer the spinach to a bowl of ice water to cool. Add the carrots to the boiling water and cook until tender, about 6 minutes. Remove the spinach from the ice water and squeeze gently to extract most of the water. Using a slotted spoon, transfer the carrots to the bowl of ice water and cool. Coarsely chop the spinach and place in a small bowl. Add 1½ tablespoons of the soy-ginger sauce and toss. Add the tuna to the remaining sauce in the bowl and toss to coat. Mix in the green onions. Let marinate at least 5 minutes. Drain the carrots.

Divide the rice between 4 bowls. Divide the carrots and spinach among the bowls, scattering over the rice. Drizzle any sauce in the bowl over. Divide the tuna among the bowls, spooning any sauce in the bowl over. Cut the avocado flesh into cubes while still attached to the skin, then scoop out the flesh and divide among the bowls. Drain the marinade from the cucumber and radishes, and then distribute the vegetables among the bowls. Sprinkle sesame seeds over everything and serve.

NOTE: *This recipe is FODMAP-friendly if you limit the avocado to ⅛ of a fruit per serving.*

Salmon Cakes with Mustard-Dill-Yogurt Sauce and Riced Cauliflower 4 SERVINGS

Based on my grandmother's original recipe, these are like crab cakes, but use convenient, affordable, and incredibly nutrient-dense canned salmon. As good cold as they are warm, salmon cakes can be batch cooked in advance and then served for lunch or dinner during the week. Riced cauliflower, available in the produce section of most markets, is a healthful alternative to rice and very tasty.

MUSTARD-DILL-YOGURT SAUCE

½ cup nonfat greek yogurt

1 tablespoon dijon mustard

2½ teaspoons minced fresh dill

¼ teaspoon sugar

¼ teaspoon cider vinegar

Coarse kosher salt

Freshly ground pepper

RICED CAULIFLOWER

1 16-ounce bag riced cauliflower

2 tablespoons extra-virgin olive oil

½ teaspoon coarse kosher salt

SALMON CAKES

2 slices fine-crumbed bread of your choice, regular or gluten-free

1 14.74- to 15-ounce can pink salmon with juices

2 large eggs, beaten to blend

½ cup plain kefir or low-fat buttermilk (see note on page 182)

1 tablespoon minced fresh dill

2 teaspoons finely grated lemon zest

¼ teaspoon baking soda

¼ teaspoon coarse kosher salt

Freshly ground pepper

Extra-virgin olive oil or canola oil for cooking

FOR THE SAUCE: Combine the yogurt, mustard, dill, sugar, and vinegar in a small bowl and stir to combine. Season to taste with salt and pepper.

FOR THE CAULIFLOWER: Preheat the oven to 400°F. Pour the cauliflower out onto a large, rimmed baking sheet. Drizzle oil over, add the salt, and stir to coat the cauliflower. Spread out on the sheet. Bake until just tender, about 12 minutes, stirring after 6 minutes. Cover to keep warm.

FOR THE SALMON CAKES: Cut the crusts from the bread, and cut the bread into 1-inch pieces. Grind in a food processor until fine crumbs form. Pour the salmon and its juices into a medium bowl. Pick out the visible bones. Add the eggs and, using a fork, mix into the salmon, breaking up the salmon until a homogenous mixture forms. Add ½ cup of the bread crumbs, kefir, dill, lemon zest, baking soda, salt, and a small amount of pepper. Mix well.

Heat a film of oil in a heavy, large skillet (preferably nonstick) over medium heat until hot. Working in batches, add the salmon mixture by ⅓ cups. Cook until golden brown on the bottom, about 3 minutes. Turn and cook until just springy to the touch and golden brown on the second side, about 3 minutes longer. Transfer to a plate and cover with foil to keep warm while cooking the remaining salmon.

Divide the cauliflower among 4 plates. Top each with 2 salmon cakes. Top each cake with a dollop of sauce and serve.

NOTE: *If you don't have kefir or buttermilk, place ½ tablespoon fresh lemon juice or vinegar into a measuring cup. Add enough low-fat milk or soy milk to measure ½ cup. Stir, and then let stand 5 minutes to thicken.*

You can make this recipe FODMAP-friendly by replacing the bed of cauliflower with actual rice, choosing plain gluten-free bread crumbs, and using lactose-free dairy products (yogurt, kefir) when called for.

White Bean and Artichoke Flatbreads 4 SERVINGS

Loaded with flavor, fibrous whole artichoke hearts and white beans become far easier for a sluggish stomach to digest when puréed to a creamy texture. This alluring Mediterranean spread makes a fine lunch staple or dip for steamed vegetables among those who aren't sensitive to higher-FODMAP foods. For quick meals, spread the purée on toasted tortillas and add toppings of your choice. My favorites are sautéed baby spinach and feta, as well as drained, jarred, roasted red bell pepper and feta.

2 tablespoons extra-virgin olive oil

1 large shallot, minced

2 teaspoons minced fresh rosemary

15.5-ounce can cannellini (white kidney) beans, drained

14-ounce can artichoke hearts (not marinated), drained, coarsely chopped

2 tablespoons fresh lemon juice

2 teaspoons grated lemon zest

Coarse kosher salt

Freshly ground pepper

8 corn tortillas

Toppings such as sautéed baby spinach; feta cheese; strips of drained, jarred, roasted red bell peppers; canned tuna; thinly sliced radishes; thinly sliced, peeled, and seeded cucumber

Heat the oil in a heavy, small skillet over low heat. Add the shallot and rosemary. Cook until the mixture is aromatic and shallot is tender, turning frequently, about 10 minutes.

Place the drained beans and chopped artichokes in a food processor. Add the shallot mixture, lemon juice, and lemon zest. Purée until very smooth. Season to taste with salt and a little pepper.

Heat the tortillas directly over a gas burner, or in a skillet or griddle over medium heat, until browned in spots on both sides. Transfer the tortillas to a work surface. Spread 3 to 4 tablespoons white bean purée over each. Add toppings of your choice. Cut each tortilla into quarters and serve.

Turkey, Bell Pepper, and Sweet Potato Hash

4 SERVINGS

If you're tired of burgers and meatballs, here's a fun alternative use for ground turkey that is low in fat but robust in flavor. This is a balanced, one-skillet meal featuring lean protein, healthy carbs, and vitamin-packed, well-softened red peppers.

> **Olive oil spray**
>
> **1¼ pounds sweet potatoes, peeled, cut into ½- to ¾-inch pieces**
>
> **1½ tablespoons extra-virgin olive oil**
>
> **1½ teaspoons smoked paprika**
>
> **Coarse kosher salt**
>
> **1 large red bell pepper, seeded, cut into ½-inch pieces**
>
> **¼ onion, minced**
>
> **1 pound ground turkey (preferably 85% lean)**
>
> **1 teaspoon minced fresh rosemary**
>
> **Freshly ground pepper**
>
> **¾ teaspoon ground cumin**
>
> **½ cup dry white wine**
>
> **2 cups chicken broth**
>
> **1 teaspoon dijon mustard**

Preheat the oven to 425°F. Spray a small, rimmed baking pan with olive oil spray. Place the sweet potatoes in a medium bowl. Add ½ tablespoon of the olive oil and toss to coat. Add ¾ teaspoon of the smoked paprika and a little salt and toss to coat. Spread the sweet potato in a single layer in the prepared pan and roast until just tender in the center, about 20 minutes.

Meanwhile, heat the remaining 1 tablespoon of olive oil in large nonstick skillet over medium-low heat. Add the bell pepper and onion and sauté for 2 minutes. Cover and cook until tender, stirring occasionally, about 10 minutes.

Increase the heat to medium-high and add the turkey and rosemary to the skillet. Sprinkle with salt and a little pepper. Cook until the turkey is no longer pink, breaking up the turkey with large spoon, about 4 minutes. Add the remaining ¾ teaspoon smoked paprika and cumin and stir until aromatic, about 30 seconds. Add the wine and boil until evaporated, about 2 minutes. Add 1½ cups of the chicken broth and simmer until almost evaporated, stirring frequently, about 8 minutes.

Stir in the sweet potatoes, remaining ½ cup broth, and mustard. Simmer until the juices are syrupy. Taste and adjust the seasonings and serve.

Grilled Fish and Zucchini Tacos with Mango-Avocado Salsa 4 SERVINGS

When clients worry that a soft-textured diet will be bland and boring, I swoop in with these flavorful fish tacos on soft corn tortillas—the perfect solution for a slow-emptying, stretch-resistant stomach. The lime-spiked salsa delivers refreshing flavor and rich avocado, without the onions and heat that can trigger acid reflux.

SALSA

1 large mango (about 14 ounces), peeled, pitted, and diced (about ½ inch)

¼ cup minced fresh cilantro

2 to 3 tablespoons (to taste) minced green onion tops (green part only)

Finely grated zest of 1 small lime

1 teaspoon fresh lime juice

1 medium avocado, peeled, pitted, diced

Coarse kosher salt

Freshly ground pepper

TACOS

¾ pound mahi-mahi or tuna

2 medium zucchini, trimmed, cut lengthwise into quarters

Olive oil

Coarse kosher salt

Freshly ground pepper

1 teaspoon ground cumin

1 teaspoon smoked paprika or paprika

Finely grated zest of 1 lime

8 corn tortillas

¾ cup (about 1 ounce) chopped baby greens (if tolerated, optional)

FOR THE SALSA: Combine the diced mango, cilantro, green onions, lime zest, and lime juice in a medium bowl. Mix. Gently stir in the avocado. Season to taste with salt and a little pepper.

FOR THE TACOS: Prepare a barbecue grill with medium-high heat.

Place the mahi-mahi and zucchini on a small baking sheet. Brush fish and zucchini on both sides with olive oil. Sprinkle with salt and a little pepper. Combine the cumin and paprika in a small bowl. Sprinkle onto both sides of fish and on the zucchini. Toss the zucchini to coat with spices. Sprinkle lime zest onto one side of fish.

Toast the tortillas briefly over a gas burner or on a griddle.

Grill the fish and zucchini until just cooked through, 4 to 5 minutes per side. Transfer to a plate. Cut the zucchini into ¾-inch pieces. Break the fish into large flakes. Divide the fish, zucchini, and salsa among the tortillas. Top with the chopped baby greens if desired, and serve right away.

NOTE: *If you don't have a grill, cook the fish and zucchini under the broiler.*

Greek-Style Braised Chicken Thighs with Olives and Red Bell Peppers 4 SERVINGS

This comforting Mediterranean dish flavored with lemon and olives satisfies without fear of reflux from garlic. Thighs rather than breasts keep the chicken moist in its flavorful juices.

1½ tablespoons extra-virgin olive oil

1½ pounds skinless, boneless chicken thighs, extra fat trimmed

Coarse kosher salt

Freshly ground pepper

¼ red onion, finely chopped

⅓ cup pitted Kalamata olives

4 strips lemon peel, removed from lemon with vegetable peeler

1½ teaspoons dried marjoram or oregano

½ cup dry white wine

½ cup chicken broth

1 cup ½-inch-wide strips roasted red bell peppers, cut from drained, jarred, roasted red bell peppers (from 12- or 16-ounce jar)

1 tablespoon fresh lemon juice

Freshly cooked white basmati or jasmine rice, or soft pita bread

Green Onion Tzatziki (see recipe, optional)

Heat the oil in a large nonstick skillet over medium heat. Sprinkle the chicken with salt and a little pepper and add to the skillet. Cook until white on the outside, about 4 minutes on each side. Transfer the chicken to a plate. Reduce the heat to medium-low, add the onion to the skillet, and cook until translucent, about 6 minutes.

Return the chicken and any juices to the skillet. Add the olives, lemon peel strips, and 1 teaspoon of the marjoram or oregano. Stir until the mixture is aromatic, about 2 minutes. Add the wine and boil for 2 minutes to evaporate the alcohol. Add the chicken broth and pepper strips. Bring to a simmer. Cover and simmer until the chicken is tender and a thermometer inserted into the thickest part registers 165°F, turning occasionally, about 30 minutes.

Uncover the skillet, add the lemon juice and remaining ½ teaspoon marjoram or oregano, and boil to reduce the liquid only slightly, 1 to 2 minutes. Season to taste with salt and a little pepper.

Spoon the chicken, sauce, olives, and bell peppers onto plates. Accompany with tzatziki, if desired, and rice or soft pita bread.

Green Onion Tzatziki MAKES ABOUT 1½ CUPS

This traditional greek yogurt–based dip is often made with loads of garlic. My version uses the digestion-friendly green onions in its place, making the dip easier on those with acid reflux and suitable for those managing bloating with a low-FODMAP diet (chapter 9).

> ½ english hothouse cucumber, peeled, seeded, coarsely grated, or finely chopped
>
> 1 cup plain nonfat greek yogurt (you may substitute plain lactose free yogurt if lactose intolerant)
>
> 2 tablespoons extra-virgin olive oil
>
> 2 tablespoons minced green onion tops (green part only)
>
> Coarse kosher salt
>
> Freshly ground pepper

Place the grated cucumber in a strainer and squeeze to remove excess liquid. Transfer the cucumber to a small bowl. Mix in the yogurt, olive oil, and green onion tops. Season to taste with salt and a little pepper. *(Can be prepared 1 day ahead. Cover and refrigerate.)*

NOTE: *Use this tzatziki to accompany grilled meats, chicken, or fish, or as a dip for broccoli steamed until soft. It is easy to grate the cucumber with a food processor.*

Vegetarian Couscous 4 (GENEROUS) SERVINGS

Moroccan-style vegetable stews—called tajines—are a traditional North African dish that are delicious when paired with couscous. Usually heavy on tomatoes, which may not be tolerated by people with acid reflux, our version offers the exotic spice flavors without the burn and vegetables that are cooked until tender. A hearty dish that isn't heavy. Make a big batch and serve once as a main course, then offer leftovers as a side dish.

2 tablespoons extra-virgin olive oil

¼ onion, finely chopped

2 teaspoons paprika

1 teaspoon ground cumin

½ teaspoon ground cinnamon

½ teaspoon ground ginger

1 15.5-ounce can organic garbanzo beans, with liquid

3 cups vegetable broth

1 pound yams, peeled, cut into 1-inch pieces (about 3 cups)

¼ cup raisins, minced

½ pound carrots, cut into ½-inch-thick rounds (about 2 cups)

1 pound zucchini, halved lengthwise, cut crosswise into ½-inch-thick pieces (about 3½ cups)

8 ounces green beans, trimmed, cut into 2-inch lengths (about 2 cups)

Coarse kosher salt

Freshly ground pepper

Freshly cooked couscous or quinoa

Chopped fresh cilantro

Heat the oil in a heavy, large pot over medium heat. Add the onion and sauté until beginning to soften, about 5 minutes. Add the paprika, cumin, cinnamon, and ginger and stir until fragrant, about 30 seconds. Add the garbanzo beans with their liquid. Simmer 5 minutes. Mash the garbanzos with a spoon. Add the vegetable broth, yams, and raisins. Increase the heat and bring to a boil. Reduce the heat, cover, and simmer 5 minutes. Add the carrots and zucchini, cover, and simmer 5 minutes. Add the green beans. Cover and simmer until the vegetables are tender, stirring occasionally, about 20 minutes. Season to taste with salt and pepper.

Spoon the cooked couscous or quinoa onto 4 plates. Spoon the vegetables and their liquid over. Sprinkle with cilantro and serve.

NOTE: *Look for organic canned beans, which tend to be softer and lower in salt than conventional.*

Southeast Asian–Flavored Baked Tofu with Shiitakes 4 SERVINGS

This is a simple-to-make, go-to weeknight recipe. Tofu is a perfectly textured protein for folks on the GI Gentle diet, but many of my patients confess that they rarely eat it since they don't know how to prepare it. Here is a great solution.

> 1 14- to 16-ounce package extra-firm tofu
>
> ¼ cup soy sauce or tamari
>
> 3 tablespoons sugar
>
> 3 tablespoons Asian fish sauce (such as nuoc mam) or soy sauce
>
> 2 tablespoons Asian (toasted) sesame oil
>
> 2 tablespoons fresh lime juice
>
> 2 tablespoons minced fresh ginger
>
> 1½ tablespoons canola oil
>
> 7 to 8 ounces fresh shiitake mushrooms, stems removed, thinly sliced
>
> Freshly cooked white basmati or jasmine rice, or quinoa
>
> Thinly sliced green onion tops (green part only)
>
> Thinly sliced fresh basil

Drain the tofu, and cut crosswise into 8 pieces. Arrange in a single layer on 2 layers of paper towels and top with 2 layers of paper towels. Let the excess water drain while preparing the marinade.

In a 7 × 11-inch glass baking dish, combine the soy sauce, sugar, fish sauce, sesame oil, lime juice, and ginger and stir until the sugar dissolves. Add the tofu in a single layer, turning to coat both sides. Let marinate about 1 hour, turning occasionally. (Can be prepared 1 day ahead.) Cover and refrigerate.

Preheat the oven to 400°F. Line a rimmed baking sheet with parchment paper. Remove the tofu from the marinade, reserving the marinade, and arrange in a single layer on the prepared sheet. Bake 20 minutes. Turn and continue baking until the edges of the tofu begins to brown, about 15 minutes longer.

Meanwhile, heat the canola oil in a medium nonstick skillet over medium heat. Add the shiitake and sauté until tender, stirring frequently, about 6 minutes. Add 2 tablespoons of water and continue cooking until the mushrooms are very tender and the water evaporates, about 30 seconds longer. Remove from the heat, add 2 tablespoons of the marinade, and toss to coat.

Spoon rice onto 4 plates. Arrange 2 tofu pieces atop each. Spoon a little marinade over each, then top with mushrooms, green onions, and basil.

NOTE: *I like to mix up the marinade in the morning, or even the night before, and then let the tofu soak. That way dinner comes together quickly.*

Butternut Squash Spoonbread 6 TO 8 SERVINGS

My family looks forward to this festive dish at all our fall holiday celebrations, and leftovers are great for lunch or brunch, topped with an egg and a sprinkle of cheese. It's easy to adapt to dairy-free and gluten-free diets by using nondairy milk and gluten-free flour. Serve it warm, spooned from the pan (hence the name), or chill overnight, cut into wedges, and reheat in the oven or microwave. It's also yummy as a snack, right from the refrigerator. Small portions should be tolerated by those on a low-FODMAP diet if you use a lactose-free milk.

> Olive oil or vegetable oil spray
>
> 2 10-ounce packages frozen butternut squash pieces
>
> 3 large eggs
>
> ½ cup all-purpose flour or all-purpose gluten-free flour
>
> ¼ cup (packed) brown sugar
>
> ¼ cup extra-virgin olive oil or canola oil
>
> ½ teaspoon coarse kosher salt
>
> 1½ cups nonfat or low-fat milk or milk substitute of your choice
>
> 1 tablespoon ground cinnamon
>
> 1 tablespoon granulated sugar

Preheat the oven to 350°F. Spray a 9-inch-diameter cake pan with 2- or 3-inch sides with olive oil spray or vegetable oil spray.

Bring ½ cup water to a boil in a heavy, medium saucepan. Add the squash. Cover and cook until the squash is very tender, about 7 minutes. Drain well. Transfer to a small bowl and mash well with a fork.

Whisk the eggs in a large bowl to blend. Add the flour and whisk until smooth. Add the brown sugar, oil, and salt and whisk until smooth. Add the milk and whisk until smooth. Add the squash and mix until blended. Pour the batter into the prepared pan.

Bake 30 minutes.

Combine the cinnamon and granulated sugar in a small bowl. Remove the pan from the oven and sprinkle the cinnamon mixture evenly over the top of the spoonbread. Return to the oven and bake until the spoonbread is puffed, feels firm to the touch, and a tester inserted in the center comes out clean, 15 to 20 minutes longer. Remove from the oven and let cool at least 20 minutes before serving. (Can be prepared 2 days ahead. Cut into wedges and reheat each piece in the microwave for about 1½ minutes, or place several wedges in a baking pan, cover with foil, and heat in a 350°F oven for about 10 minutes.)

Pub-Style Smashed Peas with Mint 4 TO 6 SERVINGS

"Mushy peas" is a classic staple of British pub cuisine, but the name hardly does justice to this creamy version. I've replaced the dried peas used in the original with frozen for a fresh flavor and emerald-green color. Whole peas can be tough on the GI Gentle diet with all of those skins, but by puréeing them, they are much more easily digested and can be a welcome addition to meals. If mint gives you reflux, just leave it out; the recipe is still divine with simple butter and salt.

> 1 16-ounce package frozen petite peas
> ½ cup water
> 1½ tablespoons butter
> 1½ teaspoons minced fresh mint
> ¼ teaspoon coarse kosher salt
> 1 tablespoon broth or water (if needed)

Combine the peas, water, and 1 tablespoon of the butter in a heavy, small saucepan. Bring to a boil. Reduce the heat and simmer until the peas are very tender, stirring occasionally, about 20 minutes.

Transfer the peas and any liquid to a food processor. Add the remaining ½ tablespoon butter and process until the peas and their skins are puréed. Mix in the mint and salt. Thin slightly with a little broth or water, if desired.

Roasted Cauliflower "Steaks" 4 SERVINGS

Center slices of cauliflower topped with bread crumbs seasoned with pine nuts, lemon zest, and fresh herbs make a beautiful and satisfying accompaniment to poultry and fish dinners. A dab of mayonnaise spread on the cauliflower helps the crumb mixture stay in place, but the recipe is still excellent without it.

> 1 large cauliflower (about 2 pounds)
> Olive oil spray
> ¼ teaspoon coarse kosher salt, plus more as needed
> Freshly ground pepper
> 1 slice fine-crumbed bread of your choice, regular or gluten-free
> 2 tablespoons pine nuts
> ¼ cup finely grated Parmesan cheese
> 1 teaspoon minced fresh thyme
> 1 teaspoon finely grated lemon zest
> 2 teaspoons extra-virgin olive oil
> 1 teaspoon mayonnaise, preferably light (optional)

Position a rack in the lower third of the oven and preheat the oven to 450°F. Line a rimmed baking sheet with parchment paper.

Remove the leaves from the cauliflower and cut the stem flush with the base; do not remove the core. Stand the cauliflower base down on a cutting board and cut 4½- to 4¾-inch-thick slices from the center of the cauliflower. Place the cauliflower slices on the prepared pan. Spray both sides with olive oil spray, and then sprinkle lightly with salt and pepper.

Roast the cauliflower until beginning to soften, about 20 minutes.

Meanwhile, tear the bread slice into 1-inch pieces. Place in a food processor and grind to fine crumbs. Transfer ½ cup of the crumbs to a small bowl. Place the pine nuts in the food processor and chop finely. Add to the crumbs. Add the cheese, thyme, lemon zest, and ¼ teaspoon salt and mix to blend. Add 2 teaspoons olive oil and toss to blend.

Spread ¼ teaspoon mayonnaise on top of each cauliflower slice, if using. Divide the crumb mixture between the slices, pressing gently to help adhere. Continue roasting until the crumbs brown, about 10 minutes. Transfer to plates and serve.

NOTE: *The recipe uses only the center slices of the cauliflower. I like to cut the remaining florets into bite-size pieces, toss them with olive oil spray, salt, pepper, and a little curry powder and then roast in a separate pan while the steaks cook. They make a great snack.*

Moroccan Spiced Carrots 4 TO 6 SERVINGS

The GI Gentle diet need not be bland. Thoughtful seasonings can deliver lots of complex flavor without reflux-provoking garlic or spiciness, as this recipe demonstrates. It is perfect as a side dish on its own, or spoon over quinoa and top with a dollop of yogurt for a comforting vegetarian lunch.

1 pound carrots, trimmed, cut diagonally into ¼-inch-thick slices

1½ tablespoons extra-virgin olive oil

1 teaspoon ground cumin

½ teaspoon ground coriander

½ teaspoon paprika

¼ teaspoon ground cinnamon

¼ teaspoon ground ginger

2 teaspoons fresh lemon juice

½ teaspoon sugar

Coarse kosher salt

Freshly ground pepper

1 tablespoon chopped fresh cilantro, parsley, or mint

Steam the carrots over boiling water until tender, about 8 minutes. Drain well.

Heat the oil in a large nonstick skillet over medium-low heat. Add the cumin, coriander, paprika, cinnamon, and ginger. Stir until fragrant, about 30 seconds. Add the carrots and stir to coat and to heat through. Mix in the lemon juice and sugar. Season to taste with salt and pepper. To serve, garnish with the fresh herbs.

Honey-and-Ginger-Poached Pears

4 TO 6 SERVINGS

This sophisticated dessert comes with added benefits: It's a total stomach soother. Behind the curtain of this French classic lies soft, low-acid pears bathed in fresh ginger to counter queasiness and honey to coat the throat. Lemon peel adds the bright citrus flavor without the troublesome acid.

> 2 cups water
>
> ½ cup honey
>
> 6 quarter-size slices peeled fresh ginger
>
> 3 long strips lemon peel, removed from the lemon with a vegetable peeler
>
> 4 medium-size firm but ripe pears (they should just give when pressed gently at the stem end), peeled, quartered, cored
>
> Nonfat greek yogurt or plain lactose-free yogurt, to serve

Combine the water, honey, ginger, and lemon peel in a medium saucepan. Bring to a simmer. Cover, reduce the heat to low, and simmer 10 minutes. Add the pears, increase the heat, and bring just to a simmer. Reduce the heat and simmer uncovered until the pears are just tender when pierced with a small, sharp knife, turning occasionally, 4 to 6 minutes.

Using a slotted spoon, transfer the pears to a bowl. Boil the liquid, ginger, and lemon peel until reduced to 1 cup, about 10 minutes. Pour the mixture over the pears. Cool slightly, then cover and refrigerate until cold, at least 2 hours. *(Can be prepared 2 days ahead. Keep refrigerated.)*

Discard the ginger and lemon peel strips. Spoon the pears and syrup into bowls. Top each with a dollop of greek yogurt and serve.

Peach-Apple Crumble for Two 2 SERVINGS

Sometimes you just crave something sweet, but having too much of a high-fat dessert lying around the house can tempt even the best of us into overdoing it. My solution is a low-fat option in a portion that's just enough to satisfy two sweet tooths. It's also great for breakfast, topped with a dollop of greek yogurt.

Vegetable oil spray

1½ cups frozen peach slices, thawed (about 1 cup when thawed)

1 apple, peeled, cut into quarters, cored, thinly sliced crosswise

¼ cup quick-cooking oats (not instant)

2 tablespoons all-purpose flour or all-purpose gluten-free flour

2 tablespoons firmly packed brown sugar

½ teaspoon ground cinnamon

¼ teaspoon ground cardamom or ginger (optional)

Pinch of salt

2 tablespoons unsalted butter, at room temperature

Preheat the oven to 350°F. Spray two 1¼-cup soufflé dishes or ramekins with nonstick vegetable oil spray. Mix the peaches and 1 cup of the apples in a medium bowl. Divide the fruit between the prepared dishes, flattening slightly. Combine the oats, flour, sugar, cinnamon, cardamom (if using), and salt in the same bowl and mix to blend. Add the butter and squeeze the dry ingredients and butter between your fingers until the mixture is crumbly. Divide among the dishes, sprinkling in an even layer.

Bake the crisps until the fruit is tender and the topping is crisp, 35 to 40 minutes. Cool slightly before serving.

NOTE: *The additives in some brands of instant oatmeal will give the crispy topping a gummy texture, so look for quick-cooking oats, or pulse rolled oats in a food processor until chopped but not powdery (about 10 pulses).*

Tropical Angel Food Sorbet Cake 12 SERVINGS

This low-fat dessert is easily assembled, not baked. It uses very-low-fat, store-bought angel food cake and naturally low-fat sorbet to create a light, tropically flavored treat that won't sit heavily in the stomach. For a pretty variation, peach and raspberry sorbets make a peach Melba–flavored dessert, or try other sorbets you love. Place sorbets in their containers in the refrigerator and let rest until just soft enough to spread atop the cake, but not melting. In my refrigerator, the mango sorbet softened in about 30 minutes, and the coconut in about an hour.

> 11-ounce rectangular angel food loaf cake
> 1¾ cups (about) mango sorbet, softened
> 1¾ cups (about) coconut sorbet, softened
> 2 to 3 tablespoons seedless berry jam

Line an 8½ × 4½-inch loaf pan with plastic wrap. Using a serrated knife, split the cake in half horizontally. Place the bottom cake layer cut side up in the prepared pan. Using a metal spoon, spread about 1¾ cups of the mango sorbet over the cake in an even layer. Pull the plastic wrap up over the sides and ends of the cake, and press gently on the sides and ends to flatten the sorbet. Freeze for 1 hour.

Using a metal spoon, spread about 1¾ cups of the coconut sorbet over the mango sorbet in an even layer. Spread the jam over the cut side of the cake top, and place the cake top over the sorbet, pressing gently to adhere. Pull the plastic wrap up over the sides and ends of the cake, and press gently on the sides and ends to flatten the sorbet. Cover with plastic wrap and freeze at least 6 hours.

Remove the plastic wrap from the frozen cake and place the cake on a platter or work surface. Trim the ends to even, if desired. Cut crosswise into slices and serve.

NOTE: *The finished dessert will keep well in the freezer for about a week.*

Chocolate-Banana Mousse 6 SERVINGS

Here's a divine, intense, dark chocolate dessert that fits the GI Gentle diet. Greek yogurt and bananas produce the signature creaminess of mousse without the fat, and high-quality chocolate delivers great flavor.

> ¾ cup nonfat milk or dairy-free alternative, such as almond milk
> 5 ounces dark chocolate, chopped
> 1½ tablespoons sugar, or more to taste
> 1 teaspoon vanilla extract
> Pinch of salt
> 2 ripe bananas, peeled, cut into large pieces
> 1 cup plain nonfat greek yogurt

Rinse out a small saucepan with cold water and drain. Add the milk and heat until bubbles form around the edges of the pan. Remove from the heat and immediately add the chocolate, 1½ tablespoons sugar, vanilla, and salt. Stir until the chocolate melts. Cool to lukewarm.

Purée the bananas in a food processor. Add the chocolate sauce and blend in. Measure the yogurt into a medium bowl. Gradually stir in the chocolate-banana mixture. Taste and add more sugar if desired. Serve or cover and refrigerate. Will keep for 5 days in the refrigerator.

NOTE: *For an equally tasty milk chocolate version, use 2 cups of greek yogurt instead of one; this will yield 8 to 10 servings.*

Low-Fat Pumpkin Spice Pillow Cookies

MAKES ABOUT 4 DOZEN

Soft cakelike cookies that are lower in fat and sugar than standard, but with great flavor. The secret is replacing some of the butter with canned pumpkin. These are wonderful on their own, even better with chocolate chips folded in. For a low-FODMAP version, use gluten-free all-purpose flour and replace the applesauce with an equivalent amount of mashed ripe banana.

> 2¼ cups all-purpose flour or all-purpose gluten-free flour
> 1½ teaspoons ground cinnamon
> 1 teaspoon baking powder
> ½ teaspoon baking soda

½ teaspoon salt

½ teaspoon ground ginger

½ teaspoon ground nutmeg

½ cup (1 stick) unsalted butter, at room temperature

½ cup firmly packed brown sugar

¾ cup granulated sugar

1 15-ounce can pumpkin

2 large eggs

1 teaspoon vanilla extract

½ cup unsweetened applesauce

1½ cups semisweet chocolate chips (optional)

Preheat the oven to 375°F. Line 2 baking sheets with parchment paper or spray with nonstick spray.

Combine the flour, cinnamon, baking powder, baking soda, salt, ginger, and nutmeg in a medium bowl. Whisk to blend.

Combine the butter and both sugars in a large bowl. Using a stand mixer or handheld beater, mix until light. Add the pumpkin, eggs, and vanilla and beat to blend. Mix in the applesauce. On low speed, beat in the dry ingredients. Beat in the chocolate chips, if using.

Drop the batter by rounded tablespoons onto the prepared pans, spacing 1½ inches apart. Bake until firm to the touch and brown on the bottoms, rotating the pans halfway through, about 18 minutes. Cool the cookies on the pans for 5 minutes. Transfer to racks and cool.

NOTE: *These keep for about 4 days at room temperature and freeze well.*

13.

The Low-FODMAP Diet

THE LOW-FODMAP DIET REDUCES STIMULATION of the gut by minimizing the amount of gas produced from indigestible carbohydrates. The diet may be helpful for you if you have certain types of bloating that originate in the intestines.

The *F* in FODMAP stands for *fermentable*, which alludes to the intestinal gassiness potential of a food. Low-FODMAP foods aren't very fermentable by gut bacteria, meaning that they're unlikely to provoke much bloat-inducing gas even if they're objectively high in fiber. The diet was developed by doctors and dietitians at Australia's Monash University, and it has revolutionized how clinicians worldwide help our patients manage certain types of bloating and the symptoms of irritable bowel syndrome (IBS) and inflammatory bowel diseases like Crohn's disease. I think back to my early days as a dietitian before I knew about the low-FODMAP diet and can't believe how on earth I managed to help my patients without it.

Meet the FODMAP Families

FODMAP is an acronym for all the types of foods that can cause excess gas in the gut. You already know what the *F* stands for, but I thought the chart below would be helpful to share so you can see what the remaining letters stand for. The *A* in FODMAP just stands for *and*.

Unless you have SIBO, it's unlikely that all of the FODMAP families will trigger bloating, gas, and generalized distress. For example, I've had patients who could eat all the GOS-rich beans in the world without gas or bloating but suffered terribly from fructans!

If you recognize one food on any of these lists that you know has given you trouble in the past, there's a good chance that other foods in that family may cause you trouble too. For example, if wheat makes you feel bloated and gassy but you don't have celiac disease, it's possible that other foods rich in fructans will give you trouble too: these include onions, garlic (and onion powder/garlic powder), artichokes, jicama, and any processed foods, supplements, or sweeteners that contain the ingredient inulin (chicory root fiber).

On the flip side, if you know you comfortably tolerate a particular food on this list, it's likely you'll do fine with the other foods in that family. If mannitol-rich cauliflower doesn't give you grief, then you're probably safe eating mushrooms, snow peas, and sugar snap peas.

Just as "location, location, location" is the first rule of real estate, so too is "dose, dose, dose" the first rule of FODMAPs. In other words, the gassiness of FODMAPs depends on how much of them you consume. For example, while wheat and onions both contain fructans, onions are a much more concentrated source of them. You may be able to get away with a modest portion of wheat—say, a slice or two of bread—without feeling much bloat, but a modest portion of onions may set off your symptoms in a significant way. Therefore, I suggest you use these lists to help narrow down which foods are most and least likely to be problematic for you, and then conduct some experiments to see whether you're able to get away with a certain portion.

If lactose turns out to be your problem FODMAP, you can take lactase enzyme supplements with lactose-rich foods to improve your

	Stands For	Includes These Families of Carbohydrates	Common Food Sources
O	Oligosaccharides	Fructans Galacto-oligosaccharides (GOS)	Fructans: 　Wheat, barley 　Onions, garlic, shallots, leeks 　Chicory root fiber/inulin 　Artichokes 　Jerusalem artichokes (sunchokes) 　Jicama GOS: 　All beans, lentils, chickpeas, peas, unfermented soybeans (and soy milk) 　Cruciferous veggies: brussels sprouts, broccoli, cabbage, kale 　Beets
D	Disaccharides	Lactose (milk sugar)	Dairy products See page 130 for a more detailed list of high-lactose dairy foods
M	Monosaccha-rides	Fructose	Certain fruits Most fruit juices and juice concentrates Honey, agave nectar Processed foods, soft drinks, and condiments sweetened with high-fructose corn syrup See page 131 for a more detailed list of high-fructose foods
P	Polyols (sugar alcohols)	Anything ending with -ol: sorbitol, xylitol, erythritol, mannitol, lactitol, etc.	Sorbitol 　Certain fruits: blackberries, apples, pears, watermelon, apricots, peaches, nectarines, plums, cherries 　Avocados (larger portions) 　Sugar-free jams/jellies, candies/confections 　Some chewable/kids' vitamins and sublingual vitamin B_{12} supplements Xylitol 　Sugar-free gum and candies Mannitol 　Mushrooms 　Cauliflower 　Snow peas and sugar snap peas 　Low-carb/low-sugar energy bars 　Some chewable enzyme supplements Erythritol 　Low sugar/diet juices and soft drinks 　Low calorie "healthy ice cream" pints 　Truvia brand sweetener

tolerance. If fructose turns out to be your problem FODMAP, an enzyme supplement called *xylose isomerase* may help improve your tolerance, though it won't help if that fructose-rich food also contains FODMAPs from other families that you're sensitive to. If GOS are your problem FOD-MAP, you can take an enzyme supplement called *alpha-galactosidase* to improve your tolerance. See chapters 9 and 14 for more details about how to use these supplements. Unfortunately, there are no enzyme supplements that improve the digestibility of polyols (sugar alcohols) or fructans.

Two-Week FODMAP Elimination Diet

If you have no idea which high-FODMAP foods are contributing to your intestinal gas and bloating, then a two-week elimination diet may be the best place to start. Two weeks is plenty of time to get your symptoms under control if FODMAPs are the issue, and once you have established a flat-belly baseline, you can begin challenging each FODMAP family, one at a time, to isolate the offending carbs.

During this elimination period, I caution you to avoid thinking about high-FODMAP foods as "bad" or "unhealthy," as many of my patients are prone to doing. Some of the healthiest foods in the world are the highest in FODMAPs, and some of the least healthy (potato chips come to mind) are low FODMAP. A food's FODMAP status is only an indication of its gassiness potential, not of its nutritional quality. The reason I mention this is because a strict, low-FODMAP diet may not be the healthiest diet to follow for the very long term, and the diet's creators consistently encourage followers not to get stuck in the elimination phase but rather to continue on to the rechallenge phase.

Many of my patients with bloating that originates in the intestines feel so wonderful after a week or two on the low-FODMAP diet that they avoid testing the boundaries of their food tolerance for fear that the bloating will return. While it can be tempting to bask in the delight of a de-bloated belly after suffering for years, try not to let that hold you back from rechallenging each family to isolate your individual triggers. Remember: You can always revert to a stricter version of the diet if needed. My goal for you is to consume the healthiest, least-restricted diet that you can comfortably tolerate.

While the low-FODMAP diet may be tricky to get used to in the beginning, the nice thing about it is that it does not require you to eliminate any entire food groups. There are low-FODMAP fruits, veggies, grains, dairy foods, and plant-based proteins to choose from in addition to all animal proteins.

Fruits

The best-tolerated fruits on a low-FODMAP diet are those low in both fructose and sugar alcohols/polyols.

Instead of these high-FODMAP fruits . . .	Try these low-FODMAP fruits instead
Apples Apricots Blackberries Cherries Figs Lychees Mangoes Nectarines Peaches Pears Persimmons Plums Pomegranates Quinces Watermelon	Bananas Blueberries Cantaloupe Clementines Coconuts Grapes Honeydew Kiwis Lemons, limes Oranges Papayas Pineapples Plantains Raspberries Rhubarb Strawberries Tangerines Tropical fruits: breadfruit, dragon fruit, guava, mangosteen, starfruit (carambola), passion fruit
Dried apples Dates Figs Goji berries Dried mangoes Prunes	Up to 1 tablespoon raisins or dried cranberries/Craisins Up to ¼ cup dried coconut (shredded or flakes)
Cranberry juice cocktail and all other fruit juices and nectars not listed on the right side of this table	100% cranberry juice diluted in water/sweetened with sugar (e.g., Simply Cranberry) Lemonade sweetened with real sugar Up to ½ cup coconut water or orange juice

Vegetables

Often when patients arrive at my office having adopted a low-FODMAP diet on their own, they complain that they've gained weight as the result of it being so carb-heavy. I'm quick to remind them that there are plenty of vegetables you can eat on a low-FODMAP diet and that most common salad ingredients are low FODMAP as well.

The trickiest part of navigating the low-FODMAP diet, however, is avoiding those veggies in the allium family: onions, garlic, shallots, and leeks. Onion powder and garlic powder are even more concentrated sources of FODMAPs than fresh. To get flavor without FODMAPs, you can use the green part of scallions (green onions), chives, and garlic

Instead of these higher-FODMAP veggies . . .	Try these low-FODMAP veggies instead
Onions (including onion powder)	Arugula
Garlic (including garlic powder)	Bamboo shoots
Shallots	Bean sprouts
Leeks	Bell peppers, chili peppers
Artichokes	Bok choy
Asparagus	Carrots
Avocados (*in portions > ⅛ of a fruit per sitting*)	Collard greens
Beets	Corn
Broccoli	Cucumber
Brussels sprouts	Eggplant
Butternut squash	Endive
Cabbage	Ginger
Cauliflower	Green beans/string beans/haricots verts
Celery	Green onions/scallions, chives, scapes (green part only)
Chayote	
Fennel bulb	Lettuce—all varieties
Jicama	Root veggies: sweet potato, white potatoes, turnips, radish, rutabaga, parsnips, celeriac
Kale	
Mushrooms	
Okra	Seaweed (Nori)
Peas	Spinach
Snow peas	Summer squash (yellow, zucchini)
Sugar snap peas	Swiss chard
Sundried tomatoes	Tomatoes (fresh)
Sunchokes/Jerusalem artichokes	Water chestnuts
Taro	Winter squash (acorn, kabocha, spaghetti, pumpkin, etc.)
Yucca	

scapes. You can also make or buy onion-, shallot-, or garlic-infused olive oils, so long as you don't eat any of the actual onion or garlic that was used to infuse it with flavor. However, you cannot use broths or stocks flavored with these veggies; the FODMAPs leach into water, but not oil.

Grains

Contrary to popular belief, the low-FODMAP diet is *not* a gluten-free diet. Some foods that contain gluten are low FODMAP, and many gluten-free grain-based products are very high in FODMAPs. Since gluten is a protein and all FODMAPs are carbs, a food's gluten content does not have any bearing on its FODMAP content. Having said that, since wheat does contain fructans, your low-FODMAP diet will probably be pretty low-wheat, but not necessarily wheat-free.

Instead of these higher-FODMAP grains . . .	Try these low-FODMAP grains instead
Unfermented wheat and flour products, including:	Sourdough bread (wheat, spelt, or rye)
Whole-wheat or white bread, rolls, pita, tortillas, wraps, or crackers	Oatmeal/oats/oat bran
Wheat berries	Quinoa
Bulgur wheat	Potato/potato starch
Pasta, macaroni, and noodles (udon, lo mein)	Rice/rice cakes/rice crackers/ cream of rice cereal
Couscous	
Cold cereals made from wheat or wheat flour	Corn/corn tortillas/tortilla chips/ grits/polenta
Farina/Cream of Wheat or Wheatena cereal	Buckwheat/kasha
Barley	Tapioca starch
Unfermented rye/pumpernickel breads	Sorghum flour
Processed and gluten-free breads, bars, or snack foods that contain:	Gluten-free breads, pastas, pizza crusts, cereals, and pancake mixes that do not contain ingredients on the left or high-FODMAP sweeteners
Inulin/chicory root fiber	
Soy flour or soy protein concentrate	
Bean flours (lentil, garbanzo, fava, etc.)	

Proteins and Dairy Foods

Only foods that contain carbs can contain FODMAPs, so all meats, poultry, fish, and eggs will be naturally free of FODMAP, unless of course they're prepared with high-FODMAP seasonings. The FODMAP

Instead of these higher-FODMAP protein foods . . .	Try these low-FODMAP proteins instead
Beans (all: black, white, kidney, pinto, etc.) Edamame (boiled soybeans) Lentils Chickpeas, hummus Split peas Soy-protein or bean-based veggie burgers Soy milk	Beef Pork Lamb Chicken Turkey Fish Shellfish Eggs Firm tofu Tempeh Miso Sunshine Burgers (Original/Garden Herb) Hemp milk, almond milk, coconut milk
Pistachios Cashews	Peanuts, peanut butter Pecans Pine nuts Macadamia nuts Walnuts Chestnuts Almonds (limit to 10 per sitting) Hazelnuts (limit to 10 per sitting) Sunflower seeds Sesame seeds Pepitas (pumpkin seeds) Hempseeds Chia seeds
Milk Yogurt and greek yogurt Buttermilk Cottage cheese Ricotta cheese Fresh mozzarella Vegan yogurt/cheese substitutes made from pea protein or cashews	Lactose-free milk Lactose-free yogurt Lactose-free cottage cheese Hard/aged cheeses: cheddar, colby, havarti, swiss, Parmesan, manchego, comte, feta, etc. American cheese Coconut yogurt
Vegan protein powders made with pea protein or soy Whey protein *concentrate*	Rice, hemp, or pumpkin seed proteins +/– low-FODMAP sweeteners Whey protein *isolate* +/– low-FODMAP sweeteners

content of dairy foods and plant-based proteins will vary, however, since these contain some carbohydrate in addition to protein.

Sweeteners, Spices, and Condiments

Processed foods, soft drinks, and condiments can be loaded with high-FODMAP ingredients that induce bloating in susceptible people. Reading labels is important! Be particularly careful when choosing foods in the following categories: granola bars/protein bars/fiber bars; protein powders; protein drinks; any packaged food labeled *low carb, sugar-free,* or *no sugar added;* reduced-calorie yogurts (e.g., 80-calorie light yogurts and 100-calorie greek yogurts); ice creams that claim to be healthy (e.g., brands that advertise 300 calories or fewer per pint); gluten-free crackers, breads, and waffles; candy, sugarless gum and mints; soft drinks and sodas.

Instead of these higher-FODMAP sweeteners and seasonings . . .	Try these low-FODMAP alternatives instead
Agave nectar	Sugar (evaporated cane juice, sucrose, table sugar, palm sugar)
Chicory root fiber	
Corn syrup solids	Acesulfame potassium
Erythritol	Aspartame
Fructose, crystalline fructose	Barley malt syrup
Fruit juice concentrates (e.g., pear juice concentrate, etc.)	Brown rice syrup
	Brown sugar
High-fructose corn syrup (HFCS)	Dextrose
Honey	Glucose
Inulin	Maple syrup (100% natural)
Invert sugar	Molasses
Lactitol	Saccharin
Lactose	Stevia (Reb-A)
Mannitol	Sucralose (Splenda)
Sorbitol	
Truvia (contains erythritol)	
Xylitol	
Yacon syrup	

Ketchup	Mustard
Salsa	Mayonnaise
Guacamole	Vinegars (all)
Pesto	Lemon/lime juice
Sriracha sauce	Worcestershire sauce
Sofrito	Fish sauce
Garlic aioli	Soy sauce
Peruvian aji amarillo paste	Oyster sauce
Marinara sauce (contains onions and garlic)	Miso paste
	Sesame oil
BBQ sauces	Tabasco brand hot sauce (original)
Commercial salad dressings	All dried spices except onion and garlic powder or blends that contain them
Broths and stocks	
Onion powder	All fresh/dried herbs
Garlic powder	Fresh chili peppers (all kinds)
Mrs. Dash seasonings	Butter
Goya adobo seasoning	All oils
Sazón Goya seasoning	
Bouillon cubes and powders	

A Sample Day on the Low-FODMAP Diet

Since all food groups are in play when you're following a low-FODMAP diet, you can also adapt the diet to your preferred style of eating, as the examples below suggest.

	Sample Plant-Based Menu	Sample Omnivore Menu	Sample Paleo-Style Menu	Sample Gluten-Free Menu
Breakfast	Plain oatmeal	Cheerios	Applegate Chicken Maple sausages	Greek omelet:
	Slivered almonds, chia seeds, or pumpkin seeds mixed in	Lactose-free milk or almond milk		Eggs
			Smoothie made with:	Spinach
		Banana or strawberries		Tomato
	Blueberries		Coconut milk	Feta cheese crumbles
	Cinnamon		Hemp protein	
			Banana	Salt/pepper
	100% natural maple syrup to taste		1 tablespoon almond butter	Serve with gluten-free crispbreads, like Le Pains des Fleurs
			Cocoa powder	

	Sample Plant-Based Menu	Sample Omnivore Menu	Sample Paleo-Style Menu	Sample Gluten-Free Menu
Lunch	Original Sunshine Burger wrapped in brown rice tortilla or Rudi's Gluten-Free Bakery plain tortilla Topped with lettuce, tomato, mustard, and/or Vegenaise Side of sweet potato fries (e.g., frozen Alexia Foods)	Tuna sandwich on sourdough bread Mayo or mustard, lettuce, tomato Side of baby carrots Grapes	Naruto-style sushi rolls (rolls wrapped in cucumber instead of rice) Sashimi pieces Pineapple and cantaloupe	Salad with any of the following ingredients: Spinach, romaine, iceberg lettuce base Carrots, cucumbers, tomatoes, peppers, corn Roasted squash Hard-boiled egg, tuna, grilled chicken Sunflower seeds 1 ounce shredded aged cheese (e.g., cheddar) Oil and vinegar or lemon juice, salt and pepper
Dinner	Firm tofu or tempeh Brown rice Stir-fry of: bok choy, pepper, carrot, green beans, bean sprouts Seasoned with ginger, scallions, soy sauce, garlic-infused olive oil, sesame seeds	Grilled chicken breast Baked potato Cooked spinach (no garlic) Garden salad (lettuce, carrots, cucumber, tomato) with red wine vinegar, olive oil, salt and pepper	Spiralized zucchini "noodles" Turkey bolognese sauce (ground turkey, crushed tomatoes, herbs, garlic-infused olive oil, red wine) Sprinkled with nutritional yeast garnish	Roasted/rotisserie chicken Quinoa Cooked green beans (butter/salt)
Snack options	Peanuts Dark chocolate Tortilla chips Berry, lemon, or chocolate sorbet sweetened with real sugar (e.g., Häagen-Dazs, Ciao Bella)	Orange or kiwis Cheddar cheese stick Rice cakes with sunflower seed butter Tate's Bake Shop gluten-free cookie (chocolate chip, ginger zinger)	Plantain chips Pumpkin seeds, walnuts, or sunflower seeds Hard-boiled eggs Coconut macaroons or meringues (made with maple syrup rather than honey)	Popcorn Original Mary's Gone Crackers Banana/peanut butter Lactose-free ice cream (e.g., Lactaid, Minus the Moo)

FODMAP Rechallenges

Assuming your bloating has responded well to two weeks on the low-FODMAP diet, it's time to rechallenge. Use table 13.1 to identify which foods are in which FODMAP family, and pick one family at a time to test. On day 1, test one "usual" portion of a food in that family at breakfast or lunch, then wait and see whether you experience any of your signature gas or bloating by bedtime. (Keep the rest of your diet low FODMAP for that day so as not to confuse the experiment.) If all's clear, then on day two, add a second portion of a food in that same family in the same sitting and see if your bloating remains well controlled by nighttime. If you pass both tests, it means that FODMAP family is probably not a problem for you, and you can move on to challenging another family. If you do well on day 1 but feel gassy and bloated on day 2, it means you have a moderate intolerance to that FODMAP family, so you should just watch portions of these foods in your diet but need not avoid them like the plague. If you're miserable and bloated even after day 1, then you've isolated a carbohydrate intolerance. Go back to your low-FODMAP diet for a few days until you feel good again, and then proceed to the next FODMAP family challenge.

Low-FODMAP Recipes

Entire cookbooks have been devoted to the low-FODMAP diet, but this curated collection should help you maximize the variety and flavor of your diet as you adjust to eating from a more limited set of foods.

BREAKFAST/BRUNCH
- Greek Frittata
- Sourdough Toast with Chard and Eggs
- Pumpkin Seed Coconut Granola (Nut-Free)
- Make-It-Your-Own Quinoa Porridge
- Creamy Polenta with Ratatouille
- Chai Chia Pudding

MAIN COURSE SOUPS AND SALADS

- Asian Niçoise-Style Salad

- Thai Beef Salad

- Low-FODMAP Broth

- Chicken Tortilla Soup

- Corn and Scallop Chowder

ENTRÉES

- Mexican Beef Bowl

- Shrimp Pad Thai

- Moroccan-Flavored Tofu Stew over Quinoa

- Pesto Pasta with Salmon and Green Beans

- Chili-Lime Chicken with Cilantro-Cumin Rice

- Tarragon and Mustard Turkey Burgers

VEGETABLE SIDES

- Roasted Kabocha Squash with Sage

- Herb-Roasted Vegetables

- Green Beans with Pecans

- Zucchini with Pesto

DESSERTS

- Citrus Salad with Cinnamon Syrup

- Coconut-Walnut Brownies

- Meringue Nests with Lime Curd and Berries

- Peanut Butter–Chocolate Chip Oatmeal Cookies

Greek Frittata 4 SERVINGS

The low-FODMAP diet need not be dairy-free; feta and Parmesan cheeses have negligible amounts of lactose and are generally well tolerated, even in the proportions here. Frittatas make a great brunch or even light supper, especially when accompanied by a salad, and the combination of melting feta cheese, sautéed red bell pepper, wilted baby spinach, and creamy eggs is lovely.

This recipe is also a good choice for people following the GI Gentle diet (chapter 12).

8 large eggs

1 cup feta cheese (about 5 ounces), crumbled, divided

¼ cup freshly grated Parmesan cheese

¼ cup thinly sliced green onion tops (green part), plus more for garnish

½ teaspoon dried oregano, crumbled

¼ teaspoon coarse kosher salt, plus more as needed

Freshly ground pepper

2 tablespoons extra-virgin olive oil

1½ red bell peppers, seeded, cut into ½-inch pieces

2 cups (packed) baby spinach leaves (about 3 ounces)

Combine the eggs, ⅔ cup of the feta, Parmesan, ¼ cup green onion tops, oregano, ¼ teaspoon salt, and a generous amount of pepper in a large bowl. Whisk to blend.

Heat 1 tablespoon of the oil in a heavy 10-inch nonstick skillet over medium heat. Add the bell pepper, sprinkle with salt and pepper, and sauté until tender, stirring occasionally, about 10 minutes. Add the spinach and stir until wilted, about 1 minute.

Add the remaining 1 tablespoon oil to the skillet, then add the egg mixture. Stir gently to distribute evenly. Reduce the heat to medium-low. Sprinkle the remaining ⅓ cup feta over the eggs. Cover and cook until the eggs are almost set but still moist in the center, about 8 minutes.

Meanwhile, preheat the broiler.

Broil the frittata until the eggs puff, the center is just springy to the touch, and the top begins to brown, about 2 minutes. Using a flexible rubber spatula, loosen the frittata around the edges. Slide onto a platter. Garnish with additional green onion tops. Serve hot, warm, or at room temperature, cutting into 4 wedges.

Sourdough Toast with Chard and Eggs 4 SERVINGS

Even better than toast and eggs, sourdough toast is topped with a pile of sautéed greens, eggs, and cheese. Contrary to common practice, the low-FODMAP diet is not a gluten-free diet (though you may use a gluten-free bread here if you avoid gluten for other reasons). Long-fermented wheat products, like sourdough breads, are naturally low in FODMAPs and are generally very well tolerated by people who find that wheat products typically bother them. For a zestier version, before adding the pepper flakes to the skillet, cook 2 garlic cloves in the oil until beginning to brown, and then discard the garlic.

4 slices sourdough bread (wheat or spelt)

3 tablespoons extra-virgin olive oil, plus more for the toast

Pinch of red pepper flakes

1 large or 2 medium bunches (1 pound total) chard, stems discarded, chopped

Coarse kosher salt

Freshly ground black pepper

¼ cup water

4 eggs

Freshly grated Parmesan cheese (optional)

Toast the bread. Brush with olive oil and keep warm in a low oven.

Heat 3 tablespoons oil in a heavy, large nonstick skillet over medium-high heat. Add the pepper flakes and cook for 20 seconds. Add the chard and sprinkle with salt and black pepper. Cook for 1 minute, stirring to coat with oil. Add ¼ cup water. Cover and cook until the chard is tender, stirring occasionally, about 5 minutes. Season to taste with salt or black pepper.

Decrease the heat to medium-low. Using a wooden spoon, make 4 indentations in the chard mixture. Break an egg into each indentation and sprinkle with salt and black pepper. Cover the pan and cook until the egg whites are set, 2 to 4 minutes. Divide the toasts among 4 plates. Using a spatula, transfer each egg with the chard around it to a toast. Sprinkle with cheese, if desired, and serve immediately.

Pumpkin Seed Coconut Granola (Nut-Free)

MAKES ABOUT 8 CUPS (ABOUT 24 ⅓-CUP SERVINGS)

This crunchy cereal is my family's obsession with its addictive balance of saltiness and just-sweet-enough-ness; I make a double batch of it every week. It's loaded with high-fiber whole grains, seeds, and coconut and light on the sugar (only 5 grams per ⅓ cup serving, or just a smidge north of one teaspoon). I've left out the nuts to keep it allergen-free and school safe; I'm guessing your kids will love it in their lunchboxes as much as mine do. Puffed millet or puffed rice adds pleasant crunch and lightness, but be certain to look for single-ingredient cereals, such as those marketed by Arrowhead Mills or Nature's Path. This is wonderful served with the milk of your choice and fresh berries.

3 cups gluten-free rolled oats

1 cup puffed millet cereal or puffed rice cereal

1 cup unsweetened coconut chips

½ cup raw sunflower seeds

½ cup raw pumpkin seeds

¼ cup (packed) brown sugar

2 teaspoons ground cinnamon

⅓ cup canola oil

¼ cup pure maple syrup (preferably dark)

2 teaspoons vanilla extract

½ teaspoon coarse kosher salt

Preheat the oven to 300°F. Combine oats, millet, coconut, sunflower seeds, pumpkin seeds, brown sugar, and cinnamon in a large bowl and mix to blend evenly. Add the oil, maple syrup, and vanilla and mix to coat the dry ingredients evenly. Mix in the salt.

Spread the granola out on a large, rimmed baking sheet. Bake until golden brown and the kitchen is perfumed with the aroma of toasting ingredients, stirring once and watching carefully to prevent coconut from over browning, about 35 minutes. Remove from the oven. Cool completely.

Transfer the granola to a covered container. The granola will remain fresh for at least a week.

Make-It-Your-Own Quinoa Porridge 4 SERVINGS

Here's a satisfying and easy-to-make alternative to oatmeal that can be cooked ahead and then reheated in the microwave. Quinoa, the base of this warming breakfast, is a highly nutritious, gluten-free seed with a slightly nutty and earthy flavor. I offer lots of tasty toppings so you can make this recipe your own. A favorite is to pour canned coconut milk over the hot cereal, then add brown sugar, blueberries, and toasted coconut.

PORRIDGE

1 cup white quinoa

1½ cups lactose-free milk, or nondairy, soy-free milk, such as coconut milk beverage or almond milk beverage

½ cup water

2 big pinches salt or to taste

½ teaspoon ground cinnamon

TOPPINGS FOR SERVING

Ground cardamom

Ground nutmeg

Butter

Nondairy, soy-free milk, such as coconut milk beverage or almond milk

Canned coconut milk

Brown sugar, sugar, maple syrup

Fresh blueberries, raspberries, or strawberries, or sliced banana

Walnuts, pecans, almonds, toasted coconut

Pumpkin seeds, sunflower seeds

Flaxseed meal, chia, hemp

FOR THE PORRIDGE: Place the quinoa in a small saucepan. Cover with about 2 inches of water, and swirl. Let stand about 2 minutes. Swirl again, and then drain well. Return the quinoa to the saucepan. Add 1 cup of lactose-free milk or nondairy milk, ½ cup water, salt, and cinnamon. Bring to a boil. Cover the pan, reduce the heat to low, and cook until the quinoa is tender and most of the liquid absorbed, about 12 minutes. Mix in remaining ½ cup milk. (Can be prepared 3 days ahead. Transfer to an airtight container and refrigerate. Before serving, spoon ¾ cups of the porridge into a microwave-safe bowl, cover, and reheat in the microwave for about 1½ minutes.)

TO SERVE: Divide the porridge among 4 bowls. Add toppings of your choice and serve.

Creamy Polenta with Ratatouille 4 SERVINGS

Try this recipe when summer vegetables are at their height. It's not time consuming to prepare because the basil and Parmesan polenta cooks in the microwave while the ratatouille simmers on the stove. Firm, blemish-free eggplants are not bitter and therefore won't need to be salted and drained before adding to the pot. Leftover ratatouille can be served with sliced sourdough baguette for an appetizer, in omelets, or as a side dish for roasted chicken or grilled fish.

This recipe is also a good choice for people following the GI Gentle diet (chapter 12).

RATATOUILLE

- 3 tablespoons extra-virgin olive oil
- 4 garlic cloves
- 1 eggplant (about 1¼ pounds), unpeeled, cut into ¾- to 1-inch pieces
- 1 pound zucchini, trimmed, cut into ¾- to 1-inch pieces
- 2 red bell peppers, stemmed, seeded, cut into ¾- to 1-inch pieces
- Coarse kosher salt
- Freshly ground pepper
- 1 pound large plum tomatoes, halved, squeezed to remove juices, chopped
- ½ cup sliced green onion tops (green part only)
- 1 tablespoon tomato paste*
- ½ cup chopped fresh basil
- 2 tablespoons red wine vinegar

POLENTA

- 4½ cups water
- 1 cup polenta (coarse cornmeal)
- 2 tablespoons extra-virgin olive oil
- 1 teaspoon coarse kosher salt
- Freshly ground pepper
- ½ cup freshly grated Parmesan cheese
- ¼ cup chopped fresh basil

FOR THE RATATOUILLE: Heat the oil in a heavy, large dutch oven over medium-low heat. Add the garlic to the pot and cook until aromatic and

---

* Look for tomato paste that does not contain honey, fructose, or high-fructose corn syrup in the ingredient list.

starting to brown, turning occasionally, about 4 minutes. Discard the garlic. Add the eggplant, zucchini, and bell peppers to the pot. Sprinkle with a generous amount of salt and pepper and sauté for 5 minutes. Mix in the tomatoes. Cover and simmer over medium heat until the vegetables are tender, stirring occasionally, about 30 minutes.

Uncover the pot, add the green onion tops and tomato paste, and simmer until the juices thicken, stirring occasionally, about 3 minutes. Mix in the basil and vinegar. Season to taste with salt and pepper.

MEANWHILE, PREPARE THE POLENTA: Combine the water, polenta, olive oil, salt, and pepper in a large microwave-safe bowl. Place in the microwave and cook at the high setting for 5 minutes. Stir thoroughly. Cook at the high setting for 5 minutes longer. Stir well. Cook at the high setting for 5 more minutes. Remove from the oven and mix in the cheese and basil.

Divide the polenta among 4 plates. Spoon the ratatouille over and serve.

Chai Chia Pudding 4 SERVINGS

Soothing and satisfying, you'll find the fragrant spices make this Indian-scented pudding hard to resist. A little canned coconut milk (not to be confused with coconut milk beverage, which is a nondairy milk substitute and is also called for in this recipe) adds welcome creaminess, and chai tea bags, available at most grocery stores, lend intriguing flavor. Made at least one night ahead, it's perfect for grab-and-go breakfasts and would also be great as a just-sweet-enough snack when the 3:00 P.M. cravings kick in. Topping each serving with any of the permitted fruits, nuts, and/or seeds adds extra nourishment. A few of the endless possibilities: oranges with almonds, bananas with walnuts, raspberries with dark chocolate chips.

> 3 chai tea bags
>
> 1 1-inch strip orange peel (orange part only)
>
> ½ cup boiling water
>
> 1½ cups (about) coconut milk beverage or other nondairy, non-soy milk substitute
>
> ½ cup canned coconut milk, well stirred
>
> 3 tablespoons pure maple syrup (preferably dark)
>
> ¼ teaspoon vanilla extract
>
> ½ cup chia seeds
>
> Cut fruit such as orange, papaya, banana, or fresh raspberries
>
> Nuts, seeds, dark chocolate chips, etc.

Place the tea bags and orange peel in a 2-cup glass measuring cup. Add ½ cup boiling water and let steep 5 minutes. Remove the tea bags and orange peel, pressing on the bags to squeeze the water into the cup. Add enough coconut milk beverage to measure 2 cups liquid. Transfer to a medium bowl and mix in coconut milk, syrup, and vanilla. Mix in the chia seeds. Let stand 5 to 8 minutes. Mix well to break up clumps of chia. Cover and refrigerate at least 4 hours or preferably overnight. (Can be made 3 days ahead. Keep refrigerated.)

Stir the pudding well and divide among 4 bowls or travel containers. Top with fruit and nuts or seeds.

Asian Niçoise-Style Salad 4 SERVINGS

Thanks to the fish, hard-boiled eggs, and potatoes, this Asian take on a classic Mediterranean salad makes a completely satisfying dinner. Balsamic vinegar might be surprising in an Asian dressing, but it is reminiscent of traditional Chinese black vinegar and is heavenly when combined with ginger and sesame oil. I like to sear fresh ahi tuna briefly, leaving the inside rare, but if you prefer fish that is cooked through, just sauté it for another minute or two on each side. Your meal will come together effortlessly if all the ingredients are ready before cooking the tuna.

1 teaspoon dijon mustard

2 tablespoons balsamic vinegar

7 tablespoons canola oil, divided

2 tablespoons Asian (toasted) sesame oil

1 tablespoon minced peeled fresh ginger

Coarse kosher salt

Freshly ground pepper

12 ounces baby Yukon Gold potatoes or baby red potatoes, halved or quartered

12 ounces green beans, trimmed

¼ cup toasted sesame seeds

1 pound ahi tuna (about 1 inch thick)

1 pound baby bok choy, sliced crosswise

1 cup cherry tomatoes, each cut in half

2 hard-boiled eggs, peeled, quartered

Place the mustard in a small bowl. Whisk in the vinegar. Gradually whisk in 6 tablespoons of the canola oil and the sesame oil. Mix in the ginger. Season the dressing to taste with salt and pepper.

Place the potatoes in a large saucepan. Add water to cover by 1 inch and sprinkle with salt. Bring to a boil and cook until the potatoes are just tender when pierced with a small, sharp knife, 12 to 15 minutes. Using a slotted spoon, transfer the potatoes to a large, shallow salad bowl. Add the green beans to the same pot and boil until just crisp-tender, about 4 minutes. Add to a bowl of ice water to stop the cooking. Drain well. Spoon 2 tablespoons dressing over the potatoes and toss to coat.

Place the sesame seeds on a small plate. Sprinkle the tuna on both sides with salt and pepper, then dip in the seeds, pressing to adhere to both sides. Heat the remaining 1 tablespoon of canola oil in a heavy, large skillet over high heat until hot. Add the tuna and sear 2 minutes on each side for very rare. Transfer to a cutting board.

Add the green beans, bok choy, and tomatoes to the bowl with the potatoes. Add ⅓ cup dressing and toss to coat. Cut the tuna into slices and arrange over the vegetables, drizzle with remaining dressing. Garnish the salad with egg quarters and serve.

Thai Beef Salad 4 SERVINGS

Thinly sliced steak, crunchy cucumbers, aromatic mint and basil, and a chili-spiked lime dressing mix together into another vivid and satisfying salad meal. By using red meat as a garnish rather than the main event on your plate, you can have the best of both worlds: a great source of iron and protein in a portion that fits into your bigger picture health goals. However, chicken breast cutlets would be equally as good. The meat is marinated while the other ingredients are prepared, and then broiled briefly, making this perfect for quick weeknight cooking.

BEEF

1 tablespoon Asian fish sauce (such as nuoc mam) or soy sauce

1 tablespoon Asian (toasted) sesame oil

1 tablespoon soy sauce

¾ teaspoon sugar

Freshly ground pepper

1 to 1¼ pound beef skirt steak, flap steak, or flank steak, cut into about 8-inch lengths

SALAD

3 tablespoons canola oil

3 tablespoons fresh lime juice

1½ to 2 serrano chilies, seeded, minced

1 tablespoon Asian fish sauce or soy sauce

¾ teaspoon sugar

Coarse kosher salt

Freshly ground pepper

1 head red leaf lettuce, torn into bite-size pieces

1 12-ounce package bean sprouts (about 4 cups)

4 persian cucumbers, halved lengthwise, and then sliced crosswise

1 cup fresh basil leaves

½ cup fresh mint leaves

⅓ cup sliced green onion tops (green part only)

3 tablespoons coarsely chopped salted roasted peanuts

FOR THE BEEF: Combine the fish sauce, sesame oil, soy sauce, sugar, and a generous amount of pepper in a small, glass baking dish. Stir until the sugar dissolves. Add the beef and turn to coat. Let marinate while preparing the salad.

FOR THE SALAD: Combine the oil, lime juice, chilies, fish sauce, and sugar in a small bowl. Season the dressing to taste with salt and pepper. Combine the lettuce, bean sprouts, cucumbers, and basil and mint leaves in a large salad bowl.

Position the oven rack so the meat will be 4 inches from the heat source, and preheat the broiler. Place the beef on a rimmed baking pan or broiler pan. Broil about 2½ minutes per side for medium-rare. Let the beef rest 5 minutes.

Add the dressing to the salad and toss to coat. Divide among 4 plates. Slice the beef thinly on a sharp angle. Divide among the plates, arranging atop the salads. Spoon any juices in the pan over the meat. Sprinkle with green onions and peanuts and serve.

Low-FODMAP Broth MAKES ABOUT 2½ QUARTS BROTH PLUS 3 TO 4 CUPS POACHED CHICKEN MEAT

When you are on the low-FODMAP diet, you're going to want an onion-less basic broth recipe for your cooking arsenal. This version can replace stock called for in any soup recipe and can also be used as a base for other savory dishes, from Thanksgiving stuffing and gravy to cooked grains or risottos. The garlic and onions are browned in oil and then discarded. This way, they add their flavor to the finished product without the undesirable fructans, which dissolve in simmering liquid but not in oil. The recipe yields a valuable bonus—lots of tender, succulent, poached chicken meat to use in soups, stews, salads, and sandwiches.

3½ to 4 pounds chicken parts (I like the family pack, which includes chicken breasts and legs)

2 tablespoons extra-virgin olive oil

4 garlic cloves

1 large onion, peeled and cut into quarters

3 quarts water

2 large carrots (unpeeled), cut into 2-inch pieces

1 cup 2-inch pieces green onion tops (green part only)

1 cup canned diced tomatoes (from 14.5-ounce can)

4 to 6 quarter-size slices peeled fresh ginger

4 parsley sprigs

3 thyme sprigs

2 bay leaves

2 teaspoons coarse kosher salt

Rinse the chicken pieces well. Heat the oil in a heavy, large pot over medium-low heat. Add the garlic and onion and sauté until fragrant and beginning to brown, stirring occasionally, about 15 minutes. Discard the onion and garlic, leaving the oil in the pot. Add the chicken and water to the pot. Bring to a boil, skimming the surface occasionally. Add the carrots, green onion tops, tomatoes, ginger, parsley, thyme, bay leaves, and salt and bring to a simmer. Cover partially and simmer slowly for 40 minutes, skimming the surface occasionally. Turn off the heat and let the chicken cool in the broth.

When the chicken is cool enough to handle, using tongs, transfer to a baking dish. Pull the skin off the chicken, and pull the meat from the bones, discarding any fat and bones. Return any juices that accumulated in the dish to the broth. Strain the broth. Cover the chicken and broth separately and refrigerate up to 4 days, or freeze.

Chicken Tortilla Soup MAKES 4 MAIN COURSE SERVINGS

Chicken soup is always popular, but this Mexican-inspired tortilla soup is irresistible. I've boosted the low-FODMAP broth recipe in this book with ancho chili powder for authentic, mild, sweet, smoky, and earthy flavors. I also use the poached chicken from the same recipe. Make the broth and chicken over the weekend, and then this becomes a perfect weeknight dinner. Don't forget to squeeze the fresh lime into the soup, and add a big handful of tortilla chips.

> 1 corn tortilla
>
> 1 14.5-ounce can diced and fire-roasted tomatoes with chilies
>
> 6 cups low-FODMAP broth (see recipe)
>
> 2 tablespoons extra-virgin olive oil
>
> 4 garlic cloves
>
> 2 tablespoons ancho chili powder
>
> ¼ teaspoon ground cumin
>
> Coarse kosher salt
>
> Freshly ground pepper
>
> 2 to 3 cups shredded cooked chicken (see recipe for low-FODMAP broth)
>
> 2 cups (packed) baby spinach
>
> Minced fresh cilantro
>
> Sliced green onion tops (green part only)
>
> Grated cheddar or jack cheese or crumbled feta cheese
>
> Fresh lime quarters
>
> Tortilla chips

Heat the tortilla directly over a gas burner or in a dry skillet over medium heat until toasted on both sides. Tear into pieces. Combine in a blender with the tomatoes and ½ cup of the broth. Purée until smooth.

Heat the oil in a heavy, large saucepan over medium-low heat. Add the garlic and cook until aromatic and starting to brown, turning occasionally, about 5 minutes. Discard the garlic. Add the chili powder and cumin, and stir until aromatic and deepened in color, about 30 seconds. Add the puréed tomato mixture and the remaining 5½ cups broth. Bring the soup to a boil, reduce the heat, and simmer until it thickens slightly and the flavors blend, about 20 minutes. Season to taste with salt and pepper.

Add the chicken to the soup and simmer until heated through, about 2 minutes. Add the spinach and simmer just until wilted, about 30 seconds. Taste and adjust the seasonings.

Ladle the soup into bowls. Sprinkle each with cilantro, green onion tops, and cheese. Serve the soup with lime wedges and tortilla chips, allowing diners to squeeze lime and crumble tortilla chips into their own soup.

Corn and Scallop Chowder MAKES 4 GENEROUS SERVINGS

Smoked paprika and coconut milk are a lighter stand-in for bacon and cream in this decadent-tasting soup. It's easy to make and uses only one pot. The scallops are succulent and are a good match for the potatoes and corn, but if you can't find scallops, salmon will be equally as tasty. Baby spinach adds great color and good nutrition too; chopped chard leaves could be used instead. Serve this lovely stew garnished with a sprinkle of green onion tops and optional prosciutto.

This recipe is also a good choice for people following the GI Gentle diet (chapter 12).

3 tablespoons extra-virgin olive oil

3 whole garlic cloves

1 red bell pepper, chopped

Coarse kosher salt

Freshly ground pepper

¾ teaspoon smoked paprika

3 8-ounce bottles clam juice

1½ pounds russet potatoes, peeled, cut into ½-inch pieces (about 4¼ cups)

1 tablespoon minced fresh thyme

1 cup canned coconut milk, well stirred

1½ cups frozen corn

1 pound bay scallops

2 cups (packed) baby spinach

2 ounces prosciutto, chopped (optional)

Sliced green onion tops (green part only)

Heat the oil in a large saucepan over medium-low heat. Add the garlic and cook until beginning to brown, turning occasionally, about 5 minutes. Discard the garlic. Add the bell pepper, sprinkle with salt and pepper, and sauté until beginning to soften, stirring occasionally, about 8 minutes. Add the paprika and stir until aromatic, about 30 seconds. Add the clam juice, potatoes, and thyme. Bring to a boil, cover partially, and simmer until the potatoes are almost tender, 10 to 12 minutes.

Add the coconut milk and corn to the pan. Simmer until the corn is tender, about 10 minutes. Add the scallops and simmer 3 minutes. Add the spinach and simmer until wilted and scallops are just opaque, about 2 minutes longer. Stir in the prosciutto, if using. Season to taste with salt (about ¾ teaspoon) and pepper.

Divide the soup among 4 large soup bowls. Sprinkle with green onion tops and serve.

Mexican Beef Bowl 4 GENEROUS SERVINGS

Who says a low-FODMAP diet has to be boring? Robust and colorful, this one-dish dinner boasts layers of intense flavors and distinct textures: fragrant jasmine rice; spiced beef enhanced with crisp-tender bell peppers, zucchini, and corn; crunchy, onion-free tomato-and-cucumber salsa; all topped with a smooth lime crema. Smoked paprika lends the smokiness of chipotles in adobo sauce without the offending ingredients. This is a meal the whole family will love.

LIME CREMA

1 cup lactose-free plain yogurt

2 tablespoons extra-virgin olive oil

1 teaspoon finely grated lime zest

Coarse kosher salt

Freshly ground black pepper

TOMATO-CUCUMBER SALSA

1 large tomato

2 persian cucumbers, trimmed, cut in ¼-inch pieces

¼ cup chopped fresh cilantro

¼ cup chopped green onion tops (green part only)

1 tablespoon fresh lime juice

½ to 1 serrano chili, seeded, minced

Coarse kosher salt

Freshly ground black pepper

BEEF AND VEGETABLES

2 tablespoons extra-virgin olive oil

1 large red bell pepper, seeded, cut into ½-inch pieces

8 ounces zucchini, trimmed, cut into ½-inch pieces

Coarse kosher salt

Freshly ground black pepper

1 pound ground beef

2 tablespoons tomato paste*

2 teaspoons smoked paprika

2 teaspoons ground cumin

½ teaspoon red pepper flakes

1½ cups corn kernels (cut from 2 ears of corn or frozen)

---

* Look for tomato paste that does not contain honey, fructose, or high-fructose corn syrup in the ingredient list.

½ cup water

1 cup brown jasmine or brown basmati rice, cooked according to package directions

FOR THE CREMA: Combine the yogurt, oil, and lime zest in a small bowl and mix to blend. Season to taste with salt and black pepper.

FOR THE SALSA: Cut the tomato in half and gently squeeze out its juices. Chop the tomato and transfer to a medium bowl. Mix in the cucumbers, cilantro, green onion, lime juice, and enough chili to season to taste. Season with salt and black pepper.

FOR THE BEEF AND VEGETABLES: Heat the oil in a heavy, large skillet over medium-low heat. Add the bell pepper and sauté until beginning to soften, about 5 minutes. Add the zucchini; sprinkle the vegetables with salt and black pepper, and sauté 2 minutes to heat through. Increase the heat to high, add the beef, sprinkle with salt and pepper, and sauté until the meat is no longer pink, breaking up the meat with the back of a fork, about 3 minutes. Add the tomato paste, paprika, cumin, and red pepper flakes and stir until aromatic, about 3 minutes. Add the corn and ½ cup water. Cook until the flavors blend and corn is just tender, stirring frequently, about 2 minutes. Season to taste with salt and pepper.

Divide the rice among 4 bowls. Top each with the beef and vegetables, a dollop of crema, and then some salsa and serve.

Shrimp Pad Thai 4 SERVINGS

The basic building blocks of restaurant pad Thai are low FODMAP—rice noodles, bean sprouts, peanuts, eggs, and shrimp or chicken—but the take-out version is typically sullied with garlic. My adaptation is just as vibrant and fresh tasting as the original, but the garlic is browned and then discarded so it fits the diet. While fish sauce and tamarind are authentic, the recipe is just as delicious when they are replaced with soy sauce or gluten-free tamari and fresh lime juice. Make certain to prepare all the ingredients before starting to cook.

For a low-carb or paleo-friendly version, make spiral-cut zucchini noodles: Use a spiral vegetable slicer to cut the outer part of 2½ pounds squash (zucchini and/or yellow summer squash) into long, thin strips (stop when you get to the seeds in the middle of the vegetables). Follow the directions below, adding the vegetable strips to the skillet after browning and discarding the garlic, and sauté until beginning to soften, about 5 minutes. Then add the bok choy, cook for 1 minute, mix in the green onion tops, and continue with the recipe. Ready-to-eat store-bought kelp noodles work well too.

This recipe is also a good choice for people following the GI Gentle diet (chapter 12).

PAD THAI

8 ounces dried flat rice noodles (pad Thai noodles)

3 tablespoons firmly packed brown sugar

2½ tablespoons Asian fish sauce (such as nuoc mam) or soy sauce

2 tablespoons soy sauce

1 serrano chili, stemmed, thinly sliced crosswise with seeds removed

1 tablespoon minced peeled fresh ginger

2 teaspoons prepared unsweetened tamarind paste or 2 table-spoons fresh lime juice

6 tablespoons canola oil

12 ounces medium or large peeled and deveined shrimp, patted dry

2 eggs, beaten to blend

3 garlic cloves

12 ounces baby bok choy, sliced crosswise ¼-inch thick

½ cup sliced green onion tops (green part only)

FOR SERVING

2 cups mung bean sprouts

½ cup coarsely chopped fresh cilantro

⅓ cup salted roasted peanuts, coarsely chopped

1 lime, cut into wedges

FOR THE PAD THAI: Place the noodles in a baking dish. Cover with very hot water and let soak until firm-tender, 20 to 30 minutes. Drain the noodles well.

Meanwhile, make the sauce by combining in a small bowl the brown sugar, fish sauce, soy sauce, serrano chili, ginger, and tamarind paste, and stir until the sugar dissolves.

Heat 1 tablespoon of the canola oil in a heavy, 12-inch nonstick skillet over medium-high heat. Add the shrimp and cook until pink and beginning to curl, about 1 minute. Transfer the shrimp to a plate. Add 2 tablespoons oil to the skillet and heat. Pour in the eggs and swirl to spread in the pan. Cook until almost set, lifting the edges to allow uncooked egg to flow under. Scramble with a wooden spoon and transfer the eggs to the plate with the shrimp.

Heat 3 tablespoons oil in the same skillet over medium-high heat. Add the garlic and cook until light brown and aromatic, about 3 minutes. Discard the garlic. Add the bok choy to the skillet and cook until slightly softened, about 1 minute. Shake the noodles to remove excess water and add to the skillet. Stir 1 minute to heat. Mix in the green onion tops. Stir the sauce to blend and add to the skillet. Gently stir the noodles until well coated, about 1 minute. Return the shrimp and eggs to the skillet and mix in.

TO SERVE: Divide the pad Thai among 4 plates. Top with bean sprouts, cilantro, and peanuts. Serve with lime wedges.

Moroccan-Flavored Tofu Stew over Quinoa

4 SERVINGS (GENEROUS)

Tofu is a soy milk–derived food whose FODMAPs have been tamed in the making. It's an essential protein staple on the low-FODMAP diet for vegetarians or those looking to eat less meat. In this Moroccan-style recipe, tofu replaces traditional— but more difficult to tolerate—chickpeas. Braising the tofu allows it to absorb the flavors of the exotically spiced tomato broth. Briefly weighting the tofu under a saucepan will help it hold together during the braising. For efficient cooking, let the tofu sit under the weight while you cut the vegetables and measure the spices.

This recipe is also a good choice for people following the GI Gentle Diet (chapter 12) if you are not prone to acid reflux from tomato-based dishes.

> 1 14-ounce package firm tofu, drained
>
> 4 tablespoons extra-virgin olive oil
>
> 1 1-pound eggplant (unpeeled) cut into ¾-inch pieces
>
> ½ pound carrots, trimmed, halved lengthwise, then cut into 1½-inch pieces
>
> Coarse kosher salt
>
> Freshly ground black pepper
>
> 2 teaspoons paprika
>
> 1 teaspoon ground cumin
>
> ½ teaspoon ground cinnamon
>
> ½ teaspoon ground ginger
>
> ¼ to ½ teaspoon red pepper flakes
>
> 2 14.5-ounce cans diced tomatoes, with juices
>
> 2½ cups water, divided
>
> ¼ cup raisins
>
> 1 cup white quinoa
>
> Chopped fresh cilantro
>
> Coarsely chopped toasted almonds

Wrap the tofu in 2 layers of paper towels. Set on a large plate. Set a heavy, small saucepan on top and let drain 20 minutes. Remove the saucepan and paper towels and cut the tofu into ½- to ¾-inch pieces.

Heat the oil in a large dutch oven over medium heat. Add the eggplant and carrots, sprinkle with salt and black pepper, and sauté 5 minutes. Add the paprika, cumin, cinnamon, ginger, and red pepper flakes and stir until fragrant, about 10 seconds. Add the tofu and stir gently to coat with spices. Add the tomatoes with their juices, 1 cup of the water, and raisins. Bring to a boil. Cover and simmer until the eggplant and carrots are tender, about 25 minutes. Season to taste with salt and black pepper.

Meanwhile, prepare the quinoa. Place the quinoa in a small saucepan. Cover with about 2 inches of water, and swirl. Let stand about 2 minutes. Swirl again and then drain well. Return the quinoa to the saucepan. Add the remaining 1½ cups water and a pinch of salt. Bring to a boil. Cover, reduce the heat to low, and cook until the water is absorbed, about 15 minutes. Turn off the heat and let stand 5 minutes. Fluff with a fork.

Divide the quinoa among 4 plates. Spoon the tofu mixture over. Garnish with cilantro and almonds and serve.

Pesto Pasta with Salmon and Green Beans

4 SERVINGS

Inspired by classic Mediterranean flavors and the healthful Mediterranean Diet, spaghetti and green beans are bathed in a zesty green pesto and then topped with gorgeous pink salmon and another dollop of the sauce. Pesto without garlic sounds virtually impossible . . . unless you know the trick. By using garlic-infused olive oil rather than whole garlic, I retain the classic pesto flavor—minus the FODMAPs. I also like this all-purpose sauce with roasted vegetables and chicken, swirled into polenta and rice, and use it in my recipe for zucchini with pesto (see recipe on page 242). It will keep for about 3 days covered tightly in the refrigerator.

LOW-FODMAP PESTO SAUCE (ABOUT 1 CUP)

½ cup extra-virgin olive oil, divided

2 garlic cloves

2 cups packed fresh basil leaves

¼ cup walnuts or pine nuts

1 teaspoon coarse kosher salt

½ cup freshly grated Parmesan cheese

Freshly ground pepper

SALMON AND PASTA

4 6-ounce salmon fillets

Extra-virgin olive oil

Coarse kosher salt

Freshly ground black pepper

8 ounces gluten-free spaghetti made from rice, corn, and/or quinoa flours, such as Barilla, Ancient Harvest, or Jovial

8 ounces green beans, trimmed, cut into 1-inch pieces

FOR THE PESTO: Combine 2 tablespoons of the oil and the peeled whole garlic cloves in a heavy, small pan over low heat. Cook until aromatic and the garlic begins to color, turning occasionally, about 8 minutes. Cool to room temperature, and then discard the garlic cloves.

Place the basil, nuts, and salt in the work bowl of a food processor and pulse to chop finely. With the machine running, add the garlic-flavored oil and remaining 6 tablespoons olive oil. Add the cheese and pulse to incorporate. Add a generous amount of pepper.

FOR THE SALMON AND PASTA: Preheat the oven to 375°F. Place the salmon on a small, rimmed baking sheet. Brush with oil and sprinkle with salt and pepper. Place the fish in the oven and bake until cooked through (just springy to the touch), about 14 minutes.

Meanwhile, add the pasta to a large pot of boiling salted water, stirring to prevent sticking. Cook for 5 minutes less than the time specified on the package, stirring occasionally, about 5 minutes for Barilla. Add the green beans, cover until the water returns to a boil, uncover, and cook until the pasta is just tender but still firm to the bite, stirring occasionally, about 5 minutes longer. Reserve ½ cup of the pasta cooking liquid. Drain the pasta and beans in a colander. Return to the same pot. Add ½ cup of the pesto and toss to coat, adding enough pasta cooking liquid by tablespoons to moisten.

Divide the pasta among 4 plates. Place 1 fish piece on each plate and spoon about 1 tablespoon pesto over each and serve.

Chili-Lime Chicken with Cilantro-Cumin Rice

4 SERVINGS

Bold flavors like ancho chilies, oregano, and coriander transform bland chicken, and cilantro and cumin spice up plain rice. Doubled, this easy recipe becomes a memorable party dish. Cutting the chicken breasts horizontally in half offers two advantages—they will cook evenly and will take just a couple of minutes grilling on each side. For the freshest flavor, don't forget to squeeze lime over the chicken before eating.

CHICKEN

3 tablespoons extra-virgin olive oil

1 tablespoon finely grated lime zest (from about 2 limes)

1 tablespoon fresh lime juice

1½ teaspoons chili powder (especially ancho)

1½ teaspoons coarse kosher salt

½ teaspoon ground coriander

½ teaspoon dried oregano, crumbled

Freshly ground pepper

4 skinless, boneless chicken breasts or 8 skinless, boneless chicken thighs (about 1½ pounds)

RICE

1 cup brown jasmine or basmati rice

1½ cups water

⅓ cup chopped fresh cilantro

2 tablespoons extra-virgin olive oil

½ teaspoon ground cumin

½ teaspoon coarse kosher salt

Freshly ground pepper

Lime wedges

FOR THE CHICKEN: Combine the oil, lime zest and juice, chili powder, salt, coriander, oregano, and a generous amount of pepper in a measuring cup or small bowl for the marinade.

Arrange one chicken breast flat on a work surface. Place palm with fingers curled back on the chicken, and using a large, sharp knife, cut in half horizontally. Repeat with the remaining chicken. (Do not cut chicken thighs in half.) Arrange half the chicken pieces in a glass baking dish.

Mix the marinade with a fork and pour half over the chicken. Turn to coat on both sides. Add the remaining chicken pieces to the dish, pour the remaining marinade over, and turn to coat both sides. Cover and refrigerate at least 6 hours or overnight.

MEANWHILE, PREPARE THE RICE: Rinse the rice and place in a heavy, medium saucepan. Add the water and bring to a boil. Cover, reduce the heat to low, and cook until the water is absorbed and the rice tender, about 25 minutes. Turn off the heat and let stand covered for 5 minutes. Fluff the rice with a fork. Stir in the cilantro, oil, cumin, salt, and pepper.

Prepare a hot fire in a gas or charcoal grill. Add the chicken to the grill. Cover and cook until just cooked through and springy to the touch, about 2 minutes on each side for chicken breasts, about 8 minutes per side for thighs. Transfer to plates. Garnish with lime wedges and serve with the rice, encouraging diners to squeeze lime over the chicken.

Tarragon and Mustard Turkey Burgers 4 SERVINGS

Juicy turkey burgers, ideal for a casual family meal, get a triple hit of great flavor from spiced-up store-bought mayonnaise; the sauce gets mixed into the coleslaw, brushed onto the bun, and slathered onto the cooked burgers. It is also great on simply cooked fish or chicken and makes an excellent salad dressing and dip for vegetables, so make a large batch to keep in the fridge to use later. While some people do okay with a little bit of cabbage on the low-FODMAP diet, I err on the side of caution and use crunchy romaine as the base for the slaw. Endive, radicchio, or arugula also work well.

TARRAGON-MUSTARD SAUCE

⅓ cup mayonnaise

3 tablespoons dijon mustard

2 tablespoons chopped green onion tops (green part only)

1 tablespoon minced fresh tarragon

1 tablespoon extra-virgin olive oil

1 teaspoon fresh lemon juice

Freshly ground pepper

ROMAINE SLAW

3 cups thinly sliced romaine heart (about 1 large)

3 tablespoons tarragon-mustard sauce

BURGERS

1¼ pounds ground dark meat turkey

¼ cup chopped green onion tops (green part only)

2 tablespoons dijon mustard

1 tablespoon minced fresh tarragon

2 tablespoons extra-virgin olive oil

¾ teaspoon coarse kosher salt

½ teaspoon freshly ground pepper

4 gluten-free or sourdough burger buns

FOR THE SAUCE: Combine the mayonnaise, mustard, green onion tops, tarragon, oil, and lemon juice in a small bowl. Mix in a generous amount of pepper.

FOR THE SLAW: Place the sliced romaine in a medium bowl. Add 3 tablespoons of the sauce and mix to coat.

FOR THE BURGERS: Combine the turkey, green onion tops, mustard, tarragon, 1 tablespoon of the oil, salt, and pepper in a large bowl. Mix gently.

Preheat the broiler. Place the buns cut side up on a baking sheet.

Heat the remaining tablespoon of oil in a heavy, large nonstick skillet over medium heat. Using wet hands, form ¼ of the turkey mixture into a ½-inch-thick patty. Place in the pan. Using your thumb, make an indentation in the center of the patty. Repeat with the remaining turkey, forming 4 patties. Cook until browned and cooked through, about 5 minutes on each side.

Meanwhile, broil buns until golden brown on cut side, watching carefully, about 2 minutes.

Place bun bottoms on plates. Spoon a little sauce onto each. Top each with a burger and another spoonful of sauce. Spoon coleslaw on top of each patty, and place the bun top over the slaw. Serve, passing any remaining slaw separately.

Roasted Kabocha Squash with Sage

4 TO 6 SERVINGS

Sweet and savory, this recipe is bound to be a winner for family dinners or on the Thanksgiving table. Squashes are among the lowest-FODMAP veggies, and kabocha and acorn are the lowest (the most popular variety—butternut—is relatively higher in FODMAP). Keep the dish simple, or dress it up with the optional fried sage leaves and roasted chestnuts. Fried sage leaves are ridiculously good, and if you haven't tried them, then you're missing out. Chestnuts, which make a festive addition, can be found roasted and peeled in vacuum-sealed bags or jars.

The squash caramelizes beautifully on an unlined, oiled baking sheet. For cleanup, pour water into the hot pan and soak briefly. For an easier version with less mess, cut each half of the squash into only 3 wedges and place skin side down in a rimmed baking pan. Brush the tops generously with the oil-syrup mixture. Roast until tender, about 1 hour. Whichever way you cook the squash, cut-up leftovers are a great addition to autumn salads, rice, or quinoa.

This recipe is also a good choice for people following the GI Gentle diet (chapter 12).

SQUASH

¼ cup extra-virgin olive oil, plus more for brushing pan

2½ to 3 pounds kabocha squash

5 to 6 ounces peeled, roasted chestnuts (optional)

¼ cup pure maple syrup (preferably dark)

2 tablespoons chopped fresh sage leaves

¾ teaspoon ground cinnamon

Coarse kosher salt

Freshly ground pepper

SAGE GARNISH (OPTIONAL)

¼ cup extra-virgin olive oil

12 to 18 whole sage leaves

Coarse kosher salt

FOR THE SQUASH: Preheat the oven to 400°F. Brush a large, rimmed baking sheet with olive oil. Using a heavy, large knife, cut the squash in half. Remove the seeds and fibers. Cut the squash into wedges that are

1-inch wide at the thickest part. Arrange cut side down on the prepared pan. Add the chestnuts to the pan. Combine the oil, syrup, chopped sage, and cinnamon in a small bowl and mix to blend. Brush the mixture over both cut sides of the squash and over the chestnuts, stirring the seasonings to blend as you work. Sprinkle the squash on both sides with salt and pepper.

Roast the squash 20 minutes. Turn the squash over and roast until tender, about 15 minutes longer.

MEANWHILE, PREPARE THE GARNISH, IF USING: Heat the oil in a small skillet over medium-high heat, until a sage leaf bubbles immediately when it is added. Reduce the heat to medium, add about 6 sage leaves, and cook until bubbling stops, 15 to 20 seconds. Using a fork, transfer to a paper towel and sprinkle with salt. Repeat with the remaining sage leaves, cooking about 6 at a time.

Transfer the squash to plates or a platter. Cut the chestnuts in halves or quarters, if desired, and sprinkle over the squash. Garnish with the sage leaves and serve.

Herb-Roasted Vegetables MAKES 4 TO 6 SERVINGS

If you're stuck following the low-FODMAP diet for a long period of time to maintain good symptom control, you'll eventually want to start pushing the limits of your basic veggie staples to keep boredom at bay. Less-common root vegetables like celeriac, rutabagas, and parsnips are all allowed, and they add different flavors and textures to your diet. They're also lower-carb stand-ins for white potatoes and other starchy root veggies, which is great if you're watching your blood sugar or weight. Use this recipe as a template, substituting sweet potatoes, red bell peppers, carrots, turnips, or acorn squash for any of the vegetables listed below— you want about 8 cups total of cut-up vegetables.

A couple of preparation tips: The skin on kabocha squash is thin, so it's not necessary to peel the vegetable. Or use a sharp vegetable peeler to remove only the peel that comes off easily. Then use a heavy, sharp knife to cut the squash in half. Scoop out the seeds and fibers, and then cut the squash into wedges, and then 1½-inch pieces. Celeriac is a little tricky to handle, but it adds unusual flavor. Use a heavy, sharp knife to cut off the top and bottom. Place cut side down on a cutting board and cut down the sides to remove the rough skin.

Nonstick vegetable oil spray (or olive oil)

½ 3-pound kabocha squash, partially peeled if desired, seeded, cut into 1½-inch pieces

½ pound rutabagas, peeled, cut into 1-inch pieces

½ pound parsnips, peeled, cut into ¾-inch-thick rounds

½ pound Yukon gold potatoes, unpeeled, cut into 1-inch pieces

1 small celeriac (celery root), peeled, cut into 1-inch pieces

4½ tablespoons extra-virgin olive oil, divided

1 tablespoon minced fresh rosemary

Coarse kosher salt and freshly ground pepper

1½ tablespoons balsamic vinegar

½ teaspoon grated lemon zest

3 tablespoons sliced green onion stems (green part only)

Position a rack in the center of the oven and preheat to 425°F. Spray large, rimmed baking sheet with nonstick spray (or brush with olive oil).

Combine squash, rutabagas, parsnips, potatoes, and celeriac (about 8 cups total) in a large bowl. Pour 3 tablespoons of oil over and toss to coat. Add the rosemary and sprinkle generously with salt and pepper; toss to coat.

Transfer the vegetables to the prepared pan. Roast until tender and brown in spots, turning occasionally, about 1 hour.

Transfer the vegetables to a serving bowl. Combine the vinegar, lemon zest, and remaining 1½ tablespoons olive oil in a small bowl. Mix to blend, pour over the vegetables, and stir to coat. Season with more salt and pepper, if desired. Sprinkle with green onion greens and serve.

Green Beans with Pecans 4 SERVINGS

Green beans almandine was once the celebration vegetable at my family holiday meals. Over the years, I've yearned for an update, and here it is. This is so easy; we enjoy it for weeknight dinners too. To trim the stem ends off the beans, pick up 6 or 8 beans, lining up their stem ends above your fist, and then simply snip off with kitchen shears. Blanch the beans whenever it is convenient, cool in ice water, and drain well. Just before serving, heat them up in the skillet with the seasonings.

> 1 pound green beans, trimmed
>
> 2 tablespoons extra-virgin olive oil
>
> ⅓ cup chopped pecans
>
> ⅓ cup sliced green onion tops (green part only)
>
> 2 teaspoons minced fresh thyme or ¾ teaspoon dried thyme or marjoram, crumbled
>
> Coarse kosher salt
>
> Freshly ground pepper

Cook the green beans in a large pot of boiling salted water until just tender, about 5 minutes. Drain. Transfer to a bowl of ice water to stop the cooking. Drain well.

Heat the oil in a heavy, large skillet over medium heat. Add the pecans and cook for 30 seconds. Add the green onion tops and cook just until fragrant, about 30 seconds. Add the beans and thyme and cook until heated through, about 2 minutes. Season to taste with salt and pepper.

Zucchini with Pesto 4 SERVINGS

Because of zucchini's mild taste, this low-FODMAP diet staple is a blank slate for many inspirations. Here, I use my ingenious garlic-free pesto to deliver bold flavors without bothering the gut. For a zucchini caprese salad, after sautéing the zucchini, layer them with slices of tomato and fresh mozzarella cheese, and then drizzle with the pesto.

> 2 tablespoons extra-virgin olive oil
>
> Pinch of red pepper flakes
>
> 2 pounds zucchini, trimmed, sliced into ¼-inch-thick rounds
>
> Coarse kosher salt
>
> Freshly ground black pepper
>
> ¼ cup low-FODMAP pesto sauce, from salmon with spaghetti, green beans, and pesto recipe, page 232

Heat the oil in a heavy, large skillet over medium-high heat. Add the red pepper flakes, then the zucchini. Sprinkle with salt and black pepper. Cook until the zucchini is just cooked through, stirring frequently, about 8 minutes. Mix in the pesto. Taste and adjust the seasoning.

Citrus Salad with Cinnamon Syrup 4 SERVINGS

Here's a perfect end to brunch, lunch, or dinner; it's quick, easy, light, and refreshing. The gently spiced syrup can also be used with any of the permitted fruits, especially tangerines, berries, pineapple, and melon. Cinnamon sticks and whole cloves add complexity to the dessert, but if you don't have them, mix ¼ teaspoon ground cinnamon and a pinch of ground cloves into the syrup after boiling.

> 6 oranges, assorted varieties (navel, blood, cara cara, etc.)
>
> 1 cup water
>
> ¼ cup (packed) brown sugar
>
> 3 whole cloves (optional)
>
> 1 2-inch cinnamon stick, or ¼ teaspoon ground cinnamon

Cut ends off oranges. Arrange one orange cut side down on a work surface, and using a small, sharp knife, cut the peel and white pith away.

Repeat with the remaining fruit. Slice the fruit into rounds and arrange on a platter.

Combine the water, sugar, cloves, and cinnamon stick in a heavy, small saucepan. Bring to a boil, stirring until the sugar dissolves. Boil until the syrup reduces to ½ cup, about 8 minutes. Remove from the heat. Pour the hot syrup over the fruit. Cover and refrigerate until ready to serve, at least 1 hour and as long as overnight.

Coconut-Walnut Brownies MAKES 12 TO 16

Rich, dark, and chocolaty, no one will suspect these brownies are gluten-free or part of a special diet. For variety, replace the walnuts with pecans or almonds, or leave off the coconut topping. Make an intriguing, somewhat healthier variation by replacing the butter with olive oil; simply mix the oil into the melted chocolate.

BROWNIES

6 ounces dark chocolate (preferably 70% to 72%), coarsely chopped

½ cup (1 stick) unsalted butter, cut into chunks

3 large eggs

1 cup sugar

1½ teaspoons vanilla extract

¾ cup brown rice flour

¼ teaspoon salt

1 cup chopped walnuts

COCONUT TOPPING

1½ tablespoons unsalted butter, cut into chunks

1¼ cups sweetened shredded coconut

⅛ teaspoon salt

FOR THE BROWNIES: Position a rack in the middle of the oven and preheat to 350°F. Line an 8-inch square glass baking dish with foil, bringing the foil up the sides of the pan.

Place the chocolate and butter in a deep metal bowl. Set the bowl in a skillet of barely simmering water. Stir occasionally until the chocolate and butter are melted and the mixture is smooth. Remove from over the water and let cool to lukewarm.

With an electric mixer, beat the eggs in a medium bowl until thick and foamy. Beat in the sugar ¼ cup at a time. Using a rubber spatula, stir in the chocolate mixture and vanilla. Add the flour and salt and mix vigorously with the rubber spatula until the batter thickens, about 40 seconds. Mix in the walnuts. Transfer the batter to the prepared pan, smoothing to even.

FOR THE COCONUT TOPPING: Place the butter in a small microwave-safe bowl. Cook in the microwave until melted, checking every 10 to 15 seconds. Mix in the coconut and salt.

Sprinkle the coconut mixture over the batter in the pan.

Bake the brownies in the middle of the oven until the coconut is golden brown, about 20 minutes. Cover the top loosely with a sheet of foil and continue baking until the brownies are just firm to the touch and a tester inserted in the center comes out almost clean, about 25 minutes longer.

Cool completely in the pan on a rack. Using the foil as an aid, remove the brownies from the pan. Cut into 12 or 16 pieces. (Can be made ahead. Cover and let stand at room temperature for up to 3 days, or wrap airtight and freeze.)

Meringue Nests with Lime Curd and Berries

MAKES 8

My cousin calls these naturally gluten-free, grain-free indulgences "clouds of deliciousness." Lime and berries are an exquisite combination, but the curd could be made with lemon instead of lime, and any low-FODMAP fruit would be welcome here. The meringues can also be baked as cookies by dropping the egg white mixture by generous tablespoons onto parchment-lined baking sheets, spacing 1½ inches apart. Bake until dry and crisp, about 1½ hours total, rotating pans from top to bottom and from front to back halfway through baking. Let cool completely in the turned-off oven. Spread any leftover curd on toasted sourdough bread for a breakfast treat.

LIME CURD
4 large eggs
½ cup (1 stick) unsalted butter, cut into ½-inch pieces
⅔ cup sugar

⅔ cup fresh-squeezed lime juice (from about 6 limes)

1 tablespoon plus 1 teaspoon finely grated lime zest

MERINGUE NESTS

¼ teaspoon ground cardamom mixed with 2 teaspoons sugar (optional)

4 large egg whites, at room temperature

¼ teaspoon cream of tartar

¾ cup sugar plus 3 tablespoons, divided

1 teaspoon vanilla extract

Pinch of salt

3 cups fresh berries (raspberries, blueberries, and/or cut fresh strawberries)

Coconut flakes, toasted (optional)

FOR THE LIME CURD: Whisk the eggs in a medium bowl. Set a fine-meshed strainer over another bowl. In a heavy-bottomed saucepan, combine the butter, sugar, lime juice, and lime zest. Cook over medium heat, stirring until the sugar dissolves, butter melts, and the mixture just comes to a simmer.

Slowly whisk the hot lime mixture into the eggs. Pour the lime-egg mixture back into the same saucepan. Cook over medium-low heat, stirring constantly, until the curd thickens enough to coat a spoon (do not boil), lifting the pan from the heat occasionally to prevent overheating, 2 to 3 minutes.

Immediately pour the curd into the strainer. Push the curd through with a rubber spatula. Let cool slightly. Cover with plastic wrap, pressing directly onto the surface of the curd to prevent a skin from forming. Refrigerate until chilled, at least 4 hours. (Can be prepared 3 days ahead. Keep refrigerated.)

FOR THE MERINGUE NESTS: Place racks in the upper and lower thirds of the oven and preheat to 200°F. Line 2 large baking sheets with parchment paper.

If using the cardamom, stir together with the 2 teaspoons sugar in a small bowl. Combine the egg whites and cream of tartar in the bowl of a stand mixer (or in a large bowl, if using a handheld mixer). Beat on medium-high speed (or high speed with the handheld mixer) until the whites hold a soft shape when the beaters are lifted, about 2 minutes. Add ¾ cup sugar 1 tablespoon at a time, beating constantly, about 1½ to 2 minutes.

Sprinkle on the cardamom mixture, if using, and add the vanilla and salt. Continue beating until the whites are stiff and glossy and hold a peak when the beater is lifted straight up, about 1 minute longer.

Dab a bit of meringue underneath the corners of the parchment papers to secure them to the baking sheets. Immediately spoon the meringue in four mounds (about ½ cup each) on each of the prepared sheets, spacing apart. Using the back of a metal spoon, gently create a wide, ¾-inch-deep well in the center of each mound.

Bake the meringues 1 hour. Rotate the baking sheets top to bottom and front to back. Continue baking until the meringues are dry, crisp, and firm, about 1 hour longer. Turn off the oven and let the meringues cool completely in the closed oven, about 2 hours. Carefully peel the meringues off the papers. (Can be prepared 3 days ahead. Store in an airtight container.)

Mix the berries and remaining 3 tablespoons sugar in a medium bowl. Let stand until juices form, about 30 minutes.

To serve, place one meringue on each plate. Spoon about 3 tablespoons of lime curd into each meringue nest. Top with the berries, sprinkle with coconut, if using, and serve.

Peanut Butter–Chocolate Chip Oatmeal Cookies MAKES ABOUT 48

Satisfying, low-FODMAP cookie-jar cookies, these make a good afternoon snack or before-bed treat. They can also deliver a tasty energy boost on hikes. If you're gluten-free, choose certified gluten-free oats, and for variety, replace the peanut butter with almond butter, the chocolate chips with chopped nuts. Convenient to keep on hand, these stay fresh for about a week in an airtight container and also freeze well.

    ¼ cup (½ stick) unsalted butter, at room temperature
    ¾ cup firmly packed brown sugar
    ¾ cup sugar
    2 large eggs
    1¼ teaspoons baking soda
    1 teaspoon ground cinnamon
    1 teaspoon vanilla extract

¼ teaspoon salt

1 cup smooth, unsalted natural peanut butter

3 cups rolled oats

1 cup semisweet chocolate chips

Preheat the oven to 350°F. Lightly butter baking sheets.

Using a standing mixer fitted with a paddle attachment or a handheld mixer, beat the butter in a large bowl until smooth. Add the brown sugar and sugar and beat until well mixed. Add the eggs, baking soda, cinnamon, vanilla, and salt and beat until smooth. Add the peanut butter and beat until smooth. Using the standing mixer or a large sturdy spoon, mix in the oats and chocolate chips.

Spoon the dough by rounded teaspoons and place on the sheets, spacing 2 inches apart. Bake until the cookies are just firm to the touch and light brown around the edges, 12 to 15 minutes. Cool 5 minutes on the sheets. Transfer to racks and cool.

A Field Guide to Digestive Support Supplements

DIETARY SUPPLEMENTS FOR DIGESTIVE HEALTH are big business. A lot of people are making a lot of money marketing remedies for abdominal pain, bloating, gas, constipation, diarrhea, improved digestion, bacterial overgrowth, and overall "gut health." As a consumer, there's a lot you should be aware of before seeking salvation in a pill.

Buyer Beware

For starters, dietary supplements are scarcely regulated by the U.S. government. Supplement marketers are not required to prove that the pills they're selling actually contain what the labels claim before placing them on a store's shelf. They're also not required to test that their products do what their marketing claims say they do. As you'd expect in an environment like this, mislabeling of dietary supplements is rampant, and false promises abound. Numerous independent audits have shown that significant proportions of herbal supplements don't actually contain any of the ingredients labeled. Others contain undeclared allergens—like wheat—that can cause adverse effects in certain people.

Even more troubling is that supplement marketers don't even have to show that their products are safe to use before they put them on a store shelf in our country. The U.S. Food and Drug Administration (FDA) typically only gets involved if enough consumers complain that a particular product caused them harm or is making false advertisements or drug-like claims. As a result, some dietary supplements are adulterated with illegal drugs like steroids or stimulants, and this can happen because many small companies rely on manufacturers in China or elsewhere abroad to manufacture their products for them. Other products can contain dangerously high levels of caffeine or hormonal gland extracts from animals whose health status is not known. Some contain potent herbal ingredients that can cause liver damage, or megadoses of certain vitamins that may cause nerve damage. A 2016 study published in the journal *Hepatology* found that one in every five cases of acute liver toxicity is caused by a dietary supplement! In my practice, I have seen this statistic come to life; multiple patients have come to me with a liver injury caused by extensive supplement regimens. Even if you believe you're purchasing products from a very reputable company, unless you've seen independent lab audits that verify your supplement contains exactly what it claims, you may be playing Russian roulette with your health.

Another thing to be aware of is that many practitioners—including medical doctors, dietitians/nutritionists, naturopaths, and chiropractors—earn money by selling you dietary supplements or referring you to particular companies that do. As a consumer, you should be aware whether a person has a personal financial incentive to steer you toward one particular treatment over another.

In this context, you can see how dietary supplement options can be a minefield to navigate. There are so many products making so many claims, even my savviest patients who take the time to do independent research struggle to know which ones might help and which ones are all hype.

When Bloating Is a Problem, a Minimalist Approach to Supplements Is Best

I don't mean to suggest that I am inherently biased against dietary supplements on principle. I'm not. While I am certainly closer to the "food first" philosophy when it comes to nutrition, there is a small toolkit of go-to supplements I *do* recommend regularly to help my patients with their digestive woes—though I do not personally sell or profit from any of them. They're inexpensive, I know them to be safe in the doses prescribed, and they generally work very well. A well-chosen supplement that's well matched to a particular problem can be life-changing for some.

But in my clinical experience, I've found that less is more when it comes to using supplements. It is rare for me to recommend more than two supplements to a patient with bloating or other digestive issues. This is because the right one or two products can generally get the job done in the context of a diet that's been tailored to your individual medical issues. Equally important, taking tons of pills is likely to make you feel worse—not better—if you have most types of bloating described in this book. Every pill has a coating and fillers of unknown effect, and a big pile of pills can slow down stomach emptying time—prolonging feelings of bloating in some and causing nausea or reflux as well. People with already slow stomach emptying (gastroparesis, or GP, chapter 3) are even at risk for developing blockages in their stomachs as the result of taking too many pills, which can clump together into an indigestible mass. At least twice per month, a patient arrives to my office on an outrageous regimen of several dozen supplement pills per day. If you have digestive problems, I can assure you that taking this many pills is part of your problem, not part of your solution.

So Many Supplements, So Little Evidence

If you've spent any time online googling around to research your symptoms, you'll surely have noticed that there are a handful of supplements that "everyone" seems to recommend for your particular digestive predicament. When you see the same supplement mentioned on multiple websites from multiple sources, it can create the illusion that this must be a well-established remedy backed by some sort of scientific evidence. Some of this impression derives from the fact that many supplements are long-standing folk remedies that have been used traditionally for generations—like peppermint, licorice root, or fennel tea for an upset stomach. But to a large extent, the reputability of many supplements is a self-generated internet phenomenon. In other words, the online echo chamber *creates* their good reputation rather than reflects an already established reputation. A well-known alternative health practitioner may post about a particular probiotic or herbal supplement as part of their protocol, and the social media community of bloggers and patients spreads the word. To an outsider stumbling upon such an online community, then, it would appear that "everyone" is in the know about this particular remedy. It lends the supplement an air of legitimacy, despite a complete lack of evidence to support its use.

Call me old-fashioned, but I try my hardest to rely on good old science to guide my decisions about whether to recommend a dietary supplement or not. I actually read those long, boring studies published in reputable journals to understand what ingredients have been tested, at what doses, for what types of problems, and with what results. When there is a lack of such scientific evidence, I look into the safety profile of certain ingredients provided by government or academic institutions to understand whether a particular product is likely to be safe to try out even in the absence of strong evidence. When supplement marketers' websites provide links to research supporting their products' usefulness, I really do click on them and review all the information provided, assessing whether it is high quality or shoddy—and whether the claims a marketer makes about their product are actually consistent with what the research concludes. (You'd be amazed how many supplement companies post links on their websites to research studies that found no benefit to using their product!)

As I was writing this book, I was pretty dismayed to see the complete absence of any research whatsoever—not just into efficacy but also into the basic safety—on many of the dietary supplements that are used casually and routinely by so many patients I encounter. In the absence of any available science to guide my recommendations, I default to the first principle of ethics that health-care providers should be bound to: "Do no harm." I consider my own clinical judgment: What have my patients' experiences—thousands over the years—been with this product? Which products have worked well—and have been well tolerated—for which conditions? Which products have harmed patients of mine in the past? Is there a reasonable expectation of safety? Are there reasonable expectations of risk? In the absence of strong scientific research, I also consider the so-called biological plausibility of its claims: Based on what we know about basic biology, is it even reasonable to imagine that this product could have an effect for a particular health condition?

The remainder of this chapter is a culmination of the analytical process described above and captures my evidence-based opinions on which dietary supplements may be most helpful for which types of digestive issues—and which ones should be avoided—as of the time of this writing. Because scientific research is constantly emerging—and this is particularly the case with regard to probiotic supplements—the information contained in this section may look slightly different in future editions of this book. That is a reflection of how knowledge of health and science evolves over time. Basing our opinions on the best available science rather than dogmatic beliefs means that we can embrace effective new remedies as they become available and walk away from those that no longer seem to hold up under scrutiny.

All supplements in this chapter are given a "bottom line" rating:

- **WORTH A TRY:** This rating is a green light. It means that there's a good (or at least decent) amount of evidence that it will be of benefit, or at least that it's got a good track record of safety such that potential benefits (if unproven) outweigh potential risks and/or that it routinely works as intended for my patients.

- **SKIP IT:** This rating is a yellow light. I use it for supplements that I think will be neither helpful nor harmful. It includes supplements with minimal to no evidence of efficacy for digestive conditions in general or bloating in particular, and a low degree of biological plausibility. Given how poorly regulated dietary supplements are, I typically err on the side of skipping such products—less is more when it comes to pills when you've got digestive troubles, remember?

- **AVOID IT:** This rating is a red light. I use it for supplements that have both minimal to no evidence of efficacy for digestive conditions and which have significant enough risks of side effects or medicine interactions that I believe the risks outweigh the potential benefits.

Some products may get a "worth a try" rating for certain conditions and a "skip it" or "avoid it" for other conditions.

Activated Charcoal: Charcoal, ash, coal

WHAT IT IS

Activated charcoal is carbon that has been heated to extreme temperatures to create tiny cracks. These cracks are able to adsorb (bind to) a wide range of organic compounds, from odor particles to medications.

WHAT MARKETERS CLAIM IT DOES

- Prevent intestinal gas and alleviate bloating.
- "Detoxify the gut" (of unspecified toxins).

WHAT IT ACTUALLY DOES

- Scientific research examining the effectiveness of activated charcoal in reducing intestinal gas is limited, and the results are conflicting.
- A few studies have shown that activated charcoal taken by mouth was effective in preventing the increase in the number of flatus events (farts) occurring after a meal high in FODMAPs. But another study failed to find any significant effect on the number of flatus events—or concentrations of hydrogen gas on the breath, which is a sign of bacterial gas production in the gut—following a meal of baked beans.
- Activated charcoal is more helpful in neutralizing the odor of your gas, though the actual amount of intestinal gas is likely to remain the same.

SAFETY AND TOLERANCE CONCERNS

- Charcoal can be very constipating. For this reason, products are often formulated with sorbitol to act as a laxative. However, the sorbitol itself can cause gas in susceptible people.
- Activated charcoal binds to organic compounds indiscriminately, and that includes your medications. It may decrease the effectiveness of certain medications (e.g., birth control, thyroid medications, antiviral drugs like protease inhibitors) if taken within several hours of each other.
- Reported side effects, which are more common in large doses, include nausea, vomiting, facial flushing, and rapid pulse.
- Activated charcoal can have blood-thinning properties, so you should not take with blood-thinning medications (warfarin/Coumadin), aspirin, or in combination with supplements like gingko, vitamin E, or high-dose fish oil.

- There is no standard dose of activated charcoal. Many products are marketed in 500 milligram doses to be taken before high-FODMAP meals.

THE BOTTOM LINE?

- Skip it. Given the underwhelming evidence that it actually reduces gas, its significant digestive tolerability issues, and the risks of drug interactions, I almost never recommend activated charcoal to my bloated patients.

Align Probiotic: Bifidobacterium infantis 35624

WHAT IT IS

Align is a probiotic supplement containing one billion colony-forming units (CFUs) of the *Bifidobacterium infantis 35624* bacteria species/strain.

WHAT MARKETERS CLAIM IT DOES

- Supports digestive regularity (regular bowel movements).
- Promotes overall digestive system health.

WHAT IT ACTUALLY DOES

- Align has mostly been studied in people suffering from irritable bowel syndrome (IBS) with abdominal pain/discomfort, bloating/distention, and irregular bowel movements. Studies have generally been very small and relied on peoples' self-reported symptom diaries.

- In two separate studies, people taking Align had greater reduction in abdominal pain or discomfort, bloating/distention, and bowel movement difficulty compared to others who were given a placebo or a different probiotic. In these studies, Align did not affect bowel movement frequency or stool consistency.

- Another study showed no difference in severity of abdominal discomfort and bloating with Align compared to placebo.

- One study conducted in people with diarrhea-predominant IBS found improvement in symptoms and stool consistency when they took a probiotic mixture containing *B. infantis* compared to those who took a placebo. But this study used a probiotic with many different bacterial strains, so it's unclear whether *B. infantis* was actually responsible for the beneficial outcome or not.

SAFETY AND TOLERANCE CONCERNS

- Like all probiotics, Align is considered very safe for most everyone except sick infants and immunocompromised people.

- The one exception in my view is among people with a history of SIBO (chapter 8), who are prone to overgrowing even "good" bacteria in their small intestines. Align and all other bacterial probiotics may "seed" the small bowel and induce a recurrence. Similarly, if you're at high risk for developing SIBO due to having low stomach acid levels from age, an autoimmune disease that decreases stomach acid levels, or use of an acid-reducing medication that ends with *-prazole,* taking bacterial probiotics may increase this risk.

- Contains milk in ingredients, so it is not appropriate for milk-allergic people.

- Increased gas and bloating may occur during the first few days of supplementation, but this generally passes.

DOSING

- 1 capsule, once daily.

- Since probiotic supplements do not colonize the colon permanently, any benefits you experience will stop within about a week of stopping use.

THE BOTTOM LINE?

- Worth a try if you are bloated in the context of IBS with constipation or irregular bowel movements. Just don't expect it to be a silver bullet. The evidence in support of Align's effectiveness for managing bloating isn't particularly high quality or strong.

- Skip it if you have a history of SIBO (chapter 8) or are at high risk for developing SIBO.

Allicin: Allium sativum, garlic extract

MAY BE SOLD AS

- AlliMed, Garlique, Kyolic

WHAT IT IS

Allicin is a garlic extract supplement that is rich in sulfur.

WHAT MARKETERS CLAIM IT DOES

- Alternative medicine practitioners claim it is an "herbal antibiotic" that can kill harmful bacteria in the gut (and treat SIBO) in lieu of prescription medications.

- Because it is illegal for supplement marketers to make "drug" claims that their products can treat or cure any disease, package labels generally do not carry any such promises.

WHAT IT ACTUALLY DOES

- Allicin has barely been studied as an antibacterial or antifungal treatment in human beings; almost all of the research has been done in labs on cells in test tubes.

- At present, there is no scientific evidence to support the claim that taking garlic extract by mouth can effectively kill bacteria in the intestines or throughout the body. In fact, despite evidence of garlic's ability to kill *Heliobacter pylori* (a bacterium that causes ulcers in the stomach) in a test tube, studies conducted in actual humans have shown limited to no antibiotic effect of allicin when studied alone or when compared to prescription antibiotics.

- There are some promising research studies that show that allicin might enhance the effectiveness of certain prescription antibiotic and antifungal medications when taken as an adjunct therapy.

SAFETY AND TOLERANCE CONCERNS

- Many studies describe adverse effects, such as abdominal pain, bloating, loss of appetite, and garlic breath.

- Large doses can cause gastrointestinal upset, heartburn, diarrhea, upset stomach, flatulence, nausea, and vomiting. Facial flushing, rapid pulse, dizziness, allergies, and insomnia have also been reported.

- It may worsen the symptoms of acute gastroenteritis (infectious diarrhea/"stomach flu").

- Garlic extract can have blood-thinning properties, so you should not take it with blood-thinning medications (warfarin/Coumadin), aspirin, or in combination with supplements like gingko, vitamin E, or high-dose fish oil.

- It may decrease the effectiveness of other drugs, including birth control drugs, cyclosporine, and antiviral protease inhibitors.

DOSING

- No dose has been established for use of allicin in treating GI symptoms due to insufficient research on the topic.

THE BOTTOM LINE?

- Skip it. Allicin is not an antibiotic and should not be taken as such. There is absolutely no scientific evidence that it effectively treats SIBO on its own or in combination with other herbal products.

- There is very limited but promising evidence that allicin could help improve the effectiveness of a prescription antibiotic. It would not be unreasonable to try using it *along with* prescription antibiotics for your SIBO so long as you tolerate it.

Aloe Vera: Aloe barbadensis

WHAT IT IS

Aloe vera is a short-stemmed, cactuslike plant with thick, fleshy leaves. The inner part of the leaf contains aloe gel and includes a compound called *acemannan*. The layer underneath the skin of the leaf contains aloe latex and includes a different set of compounds, including aloins.

WHAT MARKETERS CLAIM IT DOES

- Laxative remedy for constipation.

WHAT IT ACTUALLY DOES

- The active ingredient in aloe latex, aloin, is a stimulant that may increase contractions in the colon. It also prevents water from being reabsorbed into the body from the colon, leading to softer, more easily passed stools. Products derived from crushed whole aloe leaf will contain some latex naturally; other products that list aloe "inner leaf" as an ingredient will also have it.

- Regular use of aloe latex supplements typically leads to the development of a tolerance, requiring increased doses to maintain the laxative effect.

- Aloe gel is taken from the inner part of the aloe leaf and is not effective as a laxative. Aloe supplements sold as juice typically contain aloe gel.

SAFETY AND TOLERANCE CONCERNS

- The World Health Organization classifies whole-leaf extract of aloe vera as "possibly carcinogenic [cancer causing] to humans."

- Case reports of fatalities and severe kidney damage have been reported with high doses (1 gram per day) of aloe latex. In fact, it has been banned by the U.S. Food and Drug Administration as an over-the-counter medication ingredient due to safety concerns. (However, the ingredient remains in circulation when sold as a dietary supplement.)

- Aloe can also interact with several types of medications, including certain diuretics, heart drugs, steroids, and oral hypoglycemic agents for diabetes, causing dangerous electrolyte imbalances, or hypoglycemia.

- Pregnant women should not use aloe during pregnancy due to risks of toxicity or birth defects in the fetus.

DOSING

- There is no standard dose of aloe for gastrointestinal issues.

THE BOTTOM LINE?

- Avoid it.

- The latex portion of aloe may be effective in treating constipation, but it's potentially harmful. Aloe gel that doesn't contain latex is safe, but it also has no apparent benefit.

Alpha-Galactosidase

MAY BE SOLD AS

- Beano, Bean-zyme, Beanaid

WHAT IT IS

An enzyme derived from a species of mold called *Aspergillus niger* that breaks down a specific type of complex carbohydrate found in beans and certain vegetables.

- Prevents intestinal gas caused by indigestible carbohydrates from beans, whole grains, and certain vegetables. Taken before the first bite of problem food(s), it helps prevent gas, bloating, and discomfort.

WHAT IT ACTUALLY DOES

- Alpha-galactosidase breaks down a certain type of highly fermentable fiber (galacto-oligosaccharides, or GOS) that humans lack the enzymes to digest. By rendering this fiber digestible to humans, the enzyme prevents it from arriving intact to the colon and undergoing bacterial fermentation. This prevents the creation of excess intestinal gas from these foods.

- Research studies confirm that alpha-galactosidase taken during a meal with a sizable portion of cooked beans significantly reduced the severity of flatulence and gas-related symptoms and the number of "flatulence events" (farts) per hour compared to placebo. Both low and high doses have been shown to be effective.

SAFETY AND TOLERANCE CONCERNS

- Alpha-galactosidase is very safe for adults and children alike, except for those with a genetic metabolic condition called *galactosemia*.

- Beano brand supplements—and many other brands—are formulated with an inactive ingredient called *mannitol*. Mannitol itself is a fermentable carbohydrate and can cause gas in people sensitive to the polyol FODMAP family. The Bean-zyme brand does not contain this filler ingredient and may be better tolerated.

- It may reduce the effectiveness of the diabetes medication Precose (acarbose).

DOSING

- There seems to be a wide range of effective doses, from 240 to 1,200 GalU.

- Should be taken with the first bite of any meal containing foods with GOS, including lentils, beans, peas, beets, and vegetables in the cabbage family like broccoli, brussels sprouts, cabbage, and kale.

THE BOTTOM LINE?

- Worth a try for gas-related bloating that results from carbohydrate intolerances, constipation, and SIBO that is worsened by foods containing GOS.

- See page 202 for a full list of foods with GOS for which alpha-galactosidase is likely to improve your tolerance.

WHAT IT IS

Berberine is a compound found in several plant species (barberry, Oregon grape, prickly poppy, Chinese golden thread, California poppy, goldenseal, yellowroot) with a long history in traditional Chinese medicine for treating diarrhea and helping lower blood sugar in people with type 2 diabetes.

WHAT MARKETERS CLAIM IT DOES

- Alternative medicine practitioners claim it is an "herbal antibiotic" that can kill harmful bacteria in the gut (and treat hydrogen-predominant SIBO) in lieu of prescription medications.

- Because it is illegal for supplement marketers to make "drug" claims that their products can treat or cure any disease, package labels generally do not carry any such promises.

WHAT IT ACTUALLY DOES

- Berberine has not been studied in animals or humans as a treatment for SIBO, so there is no evidence at all to indicate whether it has an effect.

- The bulk of research into berberine has been conducted in mice, not humans. There is reasonably good evidence that berberine can have a significant blood-sugar lowering effect in people with type 2 diabetes.

SAFETY AND TOLERANCE CONCERNS

- There are many safety issues related to berberine.

- It can lower blood sugar on its own and amplify the effects of diabetes medications that also lower blood sugar (insulin, metformin, glimepiride, pioglitazone, and others) and increase your risk for hypoglycemia (low blood sugar). Since dosing is not standardized in dietary supplements, you may get an unpredictable blood sugar response when using berberine for this purpose or any other.

- It can lower blood pressure on its own and amplify the effects of blood pressure–lowering medications. If you have naturally low blood pressure or use such medications, berberine may cause dangerously low blood pressure levels.

- It can prevent the breakdown of many different types of commonly used drugs by inhibiting the enzymes that metabolize them. This could increase blood levels of certain drugs to a harmful degree. Such interactions may affect blood-thinning drugs, cholesterol-lowering statin drugs, certain antibiotics, blood pressure medications, sildenafil (Viagra), antidepressants and antianxiety meds, and many more.

- It can increase levels of bilirubin—a waste product from the liver—in your blood, leading to jaundice (yellowing of eyes and skin). Do not take it if you are pregnant or nursing, as elevated levels of bilirubin and bilirubin-induced brain dysfunction in infants/children can result.

- Common reported side effects include diarrhea, constipation, and abdominal pain.

DOSING

- There is no standard dose of berberine for digestive issues.

THE BOTTOM LINE?

- Avoid it.

- Berberine is an herbal extract with many potent pharmacological effects in the body and the potential for many serious side effects in a wide range of people.

- Ironically, eradicating SIBO is *not* one of the pharmacological effects it has been shown to have. Since there is no scientific evidence suggesting it is an effective antibiotic remedy for SIBO, I've concluded that berberine's risks outweigh its benefits.

- While berberine has shown promise in helping alleviate certain types of noninfectious diarrheal conditions, there are far safer remedies for IBS-related diarrhea that I'd try first. See also: Soluble-Fiber Supplements.

Betaine HCl: Betaine hydrochloride

WHAT IT IS

Betaine HCl is an acidic form of a naturally occurring compound called *betaine*. It is not found in nature but rather is synthesized in a lab.

WHAT MARKETERS CLAIM IT DOES

- Betaine HCl is marketed to provide more hydrochloric acid in the stomach toward improving the digestibility of food.

- Paradoxically, some practitioners also recommend it to help heal ulcers and treat GERD/esophageal reflux based on their belief that having *too little* stomach acid causes ulcers and acid reflux.

WHAT IT ACTUALLY DOES

- It is not clear what, if anything, betaine HCl actually does. No scientific research exists on the efficacy of betaine HCl in treating any digestive condition at all. It has not actually been demonstrated to change the stomach's pH level—specifically, how acidic it is.

- As an aside, there is also no evidence to support the claim that reduced stomach acid levels cause symptoms of indigestion, reflux, or ulcers. (The evidence is actually to the contrary.)

- There is insufficient safety data on betaine HCl. As a result, the U.S. Food and Drug Administration prohibits its use in over-the-counter medications, stating that it "cannot be considered generally recognized as safe and effective."

- People with gastritis, ulcers, or reflux should especially avoid betaine HCl, as additional hydrochloric acid might worsen these conditions.

DOSING

- N/A. Since there is no data on its safety or efficacy, a recommended dose cannot be provided.

THE BOTTOM LINE?

- Avoid it.

- If the FDA does not recognize it as safe and there's no evidence that it acidifies the stomach or remedies any digestive problems, my conclusion is that betaine HCl's risks outweigh its benefits.

Bromelain: Ananas comosus (pineapple) extract

WHAT IT IS

Bromelain is a protein-digesting enzyme extracted from the stem and juice of pineapples. It is not the same enzyme manufactured by the human body to digest proteins.

WHAT MARKETERS CLAIM IT DOES

- Helps digest protein in the digestive tract.

WHAT IT ACTUALLY DOES

- Bromelain has been studied in people with a few types of mild inflammatory conditions, specifically sinusitis and sports injuries. There is a very small amount of evidence that it might be helpful in reducing swelling and speeding healing from these conditions, but all research was conducted using specially coated tablets to prevent the bromelain itself from being digested in the stomach. Most dietary supplements do not have this so-called enteric coating.

- Bromelain has not been studied for a potential role as a human digestive aid. It is therefore not clear what effect, if any, bromelain has on digestive symptoms or nutrient absorption.

SAFETY AND TOLERANCE CONCERNS

- People with an allergy to pineapple, latex, wheat, celery, papain, carrot, fennel, cypress pollen, or grass pollen may be allergic to bromelain.

- Bromelain may have a mild blood-thinning effect, so you should not take it with blood-thinning medications (warfarin/Coumadin), aspirin, or in combination with supplements like gingko, vitamin E, or high-dose fish oil.

- It may also amplify the effects of certain medications (amoxicillin, tetracycline), sedative medications, tricyclic antidepressants, sleep aids, and anti-seizure medications.

DOSING

- 45,000 PU is the maximum dose per serving one should consume in a sitting according to guidelines by Health Canada. (The U.S. government does not issue guidelines.)

THE BOTTOM LINE?

- Skip it.

- It's not likely to help your bloating, though it's also not likely to hurt you so long as you don't take any of the medications listed above that might interact with it.

- I personally don't recommend it to my patients based on the lack of evidence and the fact that protease (protein digesting enzyme) deficiency isn't likely a bloated person's problem; if it were, then they'd need a more standardized preparation of animal-derived pancreatic enzyme replacement therapy anyway (see chapter 13).

Calcium Carbonate (Chewable)

COMMONLY MARKETED AS

- TUMS, Rolaids, Chooz (calcium carbonate gum)

WHAT IT IS

An uncoated, chewable, over-the-counter calcium supplement that buffers (helps neutralize) stomach acid so that any esophageal reflux you experience after a meal will be less painful and damaging.

WHAT MARKETERS CLAIM IT DOES

- "Relieves heartburn, sour stomach, acid indigestion, and upset stomach associated with these symptoms."

- Neutralizes gastric acid in the esophagus and stomach and begins working instantly.

WHAT IT ACTUALLY DOES

- Controlled studies have verified the effectiveness of calcium carbonate antacids in managing heartburn and reducing the exposure of the esophagus to acid.

- Antacids work rapidly by partially neutralizing the stomach's hydrochloric acid (raising the pH level to make it less acidic).

SAFETY AND TOLERANCE CONCERNS

- Excessive doses taken for long periods of time may cause nausea and/or vomiting, abdominal pain, bloating, constipation, and flatulence.

- Calcium supplements may increase the risk of kidney stones in people who have a history of the condition or a predisposition to them.

- Reducing stomach acid levels may interfere with the ability of certain prescription medications to dissolve or certain other vitamins to be absorbed (iron, B_{12}).

- Because the effect of calcium carbonate antacids only lasts for about 30–60 minutes, this side effect can easily be managed by separating antacids from other medications and supplements by an hour.

DOSING

- Most products range from 500 to 1,000 milligrams of calcium carbonate per chewable tablet (0.5–1 grams).

- Start with 500 milligrams per dose, and take it right before the expected onset of sour stomach symptoms (e.g., before eating a meal that usually gives you heartburn or before drinking alcohol) or immediately after symptoms set in. You can take them three times daily before main meals if needed.

- Do not exceed 7 grams (7,000 milligrams) per day.

THE BOTTOM LINE?

- Worth a try for sour stomach bloating from classic indigestion. It's a cheap, effective remedy for sour stomach bloating.

- In my experience, antacids work best when taken as a preventive measure before symptoms kick in. If you are prone to sour stomach bloating, try chewing a calcium carbonate anytime you're about to eat after having gone too long between meals or before eating a larger and/or higher-fat meal that has triggered indigestion before.

Culturelle Probiotic: Lactobacillus rhamnosus GG + inulin

WHAT IT IS

Culturelle is a probiotic supplement containing ten billion colony forming units (CFUs) of *Lactobacillus rhamnosus* GG ATCC 53103, a specific strain of bacteria occurring naturally in the human digestive tract. It also contains a prebiotic fiber called *inulin* to help feed beneficial bacteria and foster their growth.

WHAT MARKETERS CLAIM IT DOES

- "Helps with occasional digestive upset, including diarrhea, gas, and bloating."

- "Helps your digestive system work better."

- "Minimize travel-associated stomach and digestive issues."

- Culturelle has been demonstrated to be most effective in reducing the severity of diarrhea from a variety of causes, including traveler's diarrhea, antibiotic-associated diarrhea (AAD), and infection with *Clostridium difficile* (*C. diff*).

- The best evidence of Culturelle's benefit is for children with antibiotic-associated diarrhea (AAD). There is reasonably good evidence to suggest that Culturelle and other probiotics with various strains of *L. rhamnosus* bacteria may be helpful in preventing or reducing the severity of diarrhea as a side effect of antibiotic medications.

- The single, very small study investigating *L. rhamnosus* GG's effect on bloating in people with irritable bowel syndrome (IBS) did not show any benefit compared to placebo.

SAFETY AND TOLERANCE CONCERNS

- Like all probiotics, Culturelle is considered very safe for most everyone except sick infants and immunocompromised people.

- The one exception is among people with a history of SIBO (chapter 8), who are prone to overgrowing even "good" bacteria in their small intestines; Culturelle and all other bacterial probiotics may "seed" the small bowel and induce a recurrence. Similarly, if you're at high risk for developing SIBO due to having low stomach acid levels from age, an autoimmune disease that decreases stomach acid levels, or use of an acid-reducing medication that ends with *-prazole,* taking bacterial probiotics may increase this risk.

- Contains inulin as an ingredient, which is a high-FODMAP (gas-producing) type of fiber. If you are sensitive to FODMAPs in the fructan family (see page 202) or suffer from lots of excess gas to begin with, Culturelle may aggravate your symptoms.

- For everyone else, increased gas and bloating may occur during the first few days of supplementation, but this generally passes.

DOSING

- One capsule, once daily.

- Since probiotic supplements do not colonize the colon permanently, any benefits you experience will stop within about a week of stopping use.

THE BOTTOM LINE?

- Skip it for management of bloating. There's minimal evidence to support Culturelle's usefulness in managing bloating or constipation, and its formulation with inulin is likely to aggravate gas and bloating in some.

- May be worth a try if you have diarrhea-predominant IBS, acute diarrhea from an infection, a history of *C. diff* infection, or diarrhea as a side effect from antibiotics. If you have a history of SIBO (chapter 8) or are at high risk for developing SIBO, I'd skip it and choose a yeast-based probiotic instead (see: Florastor).

Deglycyrrhizinated Licorice (DGL)

WHAT IT IS

Deglycyrrhizinated licorice, also known as DGL, is a compound that is refined from the root of the licorice plant. When it is refined, the glycyrrhizin part of the plant is removed. This chemical component is associated with potentially serious side effects of high blood pressure and edema (excess fluid retention). Therefore, DGL is far safer than unmodified, whole licorice root products.

WHAT MARKETERS CLAIM IT DOES

- "Helps soothe stomach lining" (e.g., for gastritis, heartburn, acid indigestion, or gastric ulcers).

WHAT IT ACTUALLY DOES

- It's not clear what DGL actually does in the stomach. The glycyrrhizin component of licorice root seems to have an effect on the mucous cells that line the stomach, causing them to secrete more of a protective mucus coating. However, this component is removed from DGL for safety reasons.

- When studied alone as a treatment for gastric ulcers, DGL did not demonstrate any healing effect on its own or compared to a placebo.

- Some studies that tested DGL did so as part of a regimen that included an antacid, so it's not possible to know how much—if any—of the benefit came from DGL alone. Similarly, other studies have tested supplements that contained DGL in combination with other ingredients for benefit in acid indigestion and dyspepsia (see chapters 4 and 5) with some promising results, but it's impossible to know whether DGL played a role in the outcome. (For more details, see also: Iberogast.)

SAFETY AND TOLERANCE CONCERNS

- Pregnant women should avoid all forms of licorice, DGL and otherwise, because of a possible increased risk of preterm labor.

- Inactive ingredients like sorbitol or mannitol are commonly used as fillers in certain brands of DGL supplements. If you are sensitive to the polyol (sugar alcohol) family of FODMAPs (see chapter 9), look for alternatives.

DOSING

- N/A; there is no standard dose for DGL for digestive issues.

THE BOTTOM LINE?

- Skip it. There's virtually no scientific evidence to support DGL's benefit in managing sour stomach bloating or other acid-related digestive woes.

- Having said that, I have had many patients over the years swear by DGL as an effective remedy for their occasional acid indigestion. Unless you're pregnant or suffer from heart disease, DGL should be safe for occasional use. So while there's no scientific evidence to earn an endorsement from me, I typically don't object when my patients with sour stomach bloating (chapter 4) want to give DGL a try instead of other remedies like calcium carbonate for episodic heartburn or indigestion.

Digestive Enzyme Supplements

WHAT THEY ARE

Digestive enzyme supplements are formulas that contain multiple different types of enzymes designed to enhance digestion of a broad array of nutrients. Typically, they include various combinations of the following ingredients:

- Starch-digesting enzymes (amylase)*
- Protein-digesting enzymes (protease,† pepsin)
- Fat-digesting enzymes (lipase‡)
- Lactose-digesting enzyme (lactase)
- Various vegetable fiber–digesting enzymes (such as alpha-galactosidase, phytases, pectinases, cellulases, hemicellulases, xylanases, typically derived from mold/fungi)
- Table sugar–digesting enzymes (invertase)
- Fruit-derived protein-digesting enzymes (bromelain and/or papain)
- Ox bile, which is a digestive fluid derived from oxen, that helps break down large fat droplets into smaller ones so that lipases can digest them more effectively
- Betaine HCl (see separate entry for more information on this ingredient)

When product labels list the source of the enzyme, *porcine* means pigs. *Aspergillus* is a type of mold and is considered a vegetarian source. *Trichoderma* is a type of fungus and is also considered a vegetarian source. Ox is exactly what you think: a male cow.

These dietary supplements are *not* the same as prescription digestive enzymes known as pancreatic enzyme replacement therapy

---

* Some products list an ingredient called pancreatin, which is a combination of amylase, protease, and lipase.
† Some products list an ingredient called pancreatin, which is a combination of amylase, protease, and lipase.
‡ Some products list an ingredient called pancreatin, which is a combination of amylase, protease, and lipase.

(PERT) used by people with cystic fibrosis or pancreatic insufficiency whose bodies do not secrete enough pancreatic enzymes. The main differences are:

- The supplement is formulated with much lower doses of amylase, protease, and lipase than the prescription version. However, a few high-potency products do have lipase levels in the same range as prescription products on the lower end of the scale.

- The supplement version is not well regulated and thus may not have standardized doses. Doses can vary from batch to batch or have higher or lower doses than those listed on the label.

- The supplement version may or may not be *enteric coated,* or coated with an acid-resistant capsule so that the enzymes survive intact until reaching the small intestine.

- The supplement contains many other enzymes besides the three pancreatic enzymes (pancreatin).

WHAT MARKETERS CLAIM IT DOES

- Supports digestion.
- Improves/promotes nutrient absorption.
- Reduces post-meal discomfort.
- Some enzyme products are marketed as "biofilm defense" products, which is code for a claim that the product helps treat and prevent SIBO. Marketers claim that their products "dissolve the sugar and fibrin components" of clumped-together bacteria that adhere to the surface of your intestines.

WHAT IT ACTUALLY DOES

- The effect of a digestive enzyme supplement will vary based on what's actually in it.

- Two very small, randomized controlled trials have examined the effects of giving healthy people lipase before a high-fat meal. Those who took the lipase reported feeling less bloating, gas, fullness, and nausea after eating compared to those who were given a placebo. However, the lipase doses used in these studies were prescription strength and significantly higher than those contained in the standard dietary supplement.

- One small study showed no benefit of prescription pancreatic enzymes on symptoms in people with functional dyspepsia (chapter 5) compared to a placebo.

- See entries for alpha-galactosidase, lactase, and xylose isomerase for a discussion of the effects of these enzyme ingredients. In short, they should be helpful in reducing gas, bloating, and/or diarrhea associated with eating beans and GOS-containing vegetables, dairy products, and high-fructose foods, respectively, among people sensitive to these foods.

- Small human studies suggest an improvement in iron absorption when a mold-derived phytase supplement is taken with a meal that contains whole grains.

- Various protein- and starch-digesting enzymes have not shown much of a benefit on digestive symptoms in people whose bodies produce enough pancreatic enzymes, though in fairness, they've barely been examined at all.

- The claim that taking any supplemental enzymes can prevent bacterial overgrowth, prevent any bacterial infection, or modify the composition of your gut's microbial ecosystem at all has no evidence to support it. And there are no biofilms in the human gut; biofilms cannot adhere to moving surfaces, such as the constantly contracting digestive tract—and this is particularly so for moving surfaces lined with a mucus layer that sheds itself every few days.

SAFETY AND TOLERANCE CONCERNS

- Digestive enzymes should generally be quite safe.

- The biggest safety issue from my perspective pertains to products that contain ox- or other bovine-derived ingredients. Any tissues or secretions that come from cows can transmit mad cow disease (bovine spongiform encephalopathy, or BSE). Given the poor regulation of dietary supplements in the United States and the likelihood that ingredients may be sourced from unknown parts of the world from animals of dubious quality, it is too risky to consume such ingredients in the absence of a known medical benefit. (There are no data supporting the benefit of ox bile supplements on human digestion.)

- Another more hypothetical safety issue with digestive enzyme cocktails pertains to excessive exposure to lipase, which can damage the colon. Very high doses of supplemental lipase can cause a scarlike thickening of the colon's walls that leads to constipation and possibly even obstructions, though admittedly, this should not be a risk with the relatively low levels of lipase contained in the dietary supplement products I've reviewed.

- On a separate note, some brands of digestive enzyme products contain prebiotic ingredients like fructo-oligosaccharides (FOS) or inulin (chicory root fiber) that may cause gas and bloating in people already predisposed to bloating.

DOSING

- Typically, product usage directions advise taking three pills daily, one with each main meal.

THE BOTTOM LINE?

- Depending on the ingredients, worth a try for post-meal bloating associated with high-fat meals or certain carbohydrate intolerances, but not particularly economical.

- While digestive enzyme cocktails contain some known-to-be-effective ingredients for people with carbohydrate intolerances, I recommend tailoring your enzyme supplement regimen to those nutrients you actually malabsorb: lactase for lactose-intolerant people, xylose isomerase for fructose-intolerant people, alpha-galactosidase for people who get too gassy from beans and broccoli. Why pay for all those enzymes you don't need? Why use a supplement that may contain too-low levels of the one or two ingredients you actually do need instead of a single-ingredient enzyme that contains a more adequate dose? Why use expensive digestive enzyme supplements routinely with all meals even if they don't contain your trigger food(s)?

- If you do decide to give them a try, I'd avoid products that contain any bovine (cow-derived) ingredients, including ox bile.

- Skip it if your goal is to use digestive enzymes to prevent SIBO.

Diatomaceous Earth

ALSO MARKETED AS

- Silica, DE

WHAT IT IS

Diatomaceous earth is a fine white powder made from ground-up rocks that are rich in a substance called *silica*. It gets its name from diatoms, the algae whose fossilized skeletons formed the sedimentary rocks from which DE is derived.

WHAT MARKETERS CLAIM IT DOES

- "Detoxify the gut" (of unspecified toxins) by trapping undesirable toxins and/or "scrubbing the walls of the intestines."

- Support healthy digestion.

- Improve absorption of nutrients.

- Regulate bowel movements.

WHAT IT ACTUALLY DOES

- Silica is mildly abrasive, and it absorbs water. It's used widely in industry for a variety of purposes: to make toothpastes slightly gritty, to filter liquids and beverages, to kill insects by dehydrating them, and to add to animal feed to absorb moisture and prevent it from clumping.

- It's literally anyone's guess as to what, if anything, silica does in the human gut other than just sit there, possibly sopping up some water. It hasn't been studied at all as a dietary supplement in humans and has barely even been studied as a supplement for animals.

SAFETY AND TOLERANCE CONCERNS

- There are numerous studies linking the inhalation of crystalline silica by diatomaceous earth workers and lung cancer. Since DE is sold in a powdered form, there may be safety concerns if the product is inhaled.

- DE is not toxic to humans when ingested and is recognized as safe by the Food and Drug Administration for use as a filter aid in food processing (e.g., to clarify wine) or when used as an ingredient in paper/cardboard used for food packaging.

- It is unclear whether DE would interfere with drug or nutrient absorption in the gut, but this is certainly a possibility and even a likelihood.

DOSING

- No standard doses exist.

THE BOTTOM LINE?

- Skip it. Silica is not an essential nutrient, and there's no evidence that it's at all beneficial to managing bloating or any other digestive conditions. Soluble-fiber supplements are a far safer way to absorb extra water in the gut if that's what you're after. And your colon does not need (or want) to be exfoliated by abrasive powdered rocks.

FDgard

WHAT IT IS

FDgard is a combination of peppermint oil (21 milligrams) and caraway (*Carum carvi*) seed oil (25 milligrams) formulated in a capsule. Caraway is a plant related to carrots that has a long history of culinary use in Europe, the Middle East, and North Africa.

WHAT MARKETERS CLAIM IT DOES

- Manage the upper-abdominal symptoms of functional dyspepsia (FD), which may include pain, discomfort, early fullness with meals, nausea, bloating, and belching.

WHAT IT ACTUALLY DOES

- The peppermint oil–caraway seed oil combo seemed to capture the attention of German researchers about fifteen to twenty years ago, and there were a handful of studies done around that time that tested this herbal remedy in patients with FD. Four randomized trials yielded statistically significant results, though only three of them were controlled with a placebo or a different medication group.

- In all of these studies, people with FD given a caraway seed oil–peppermint oil combo pill demonstrated significant symptom improvement in terms of intensity of pain, sensation of pressure, heaviness/fullness—compared to their own baseline symptoms, a placebo group, or a different medication.

- Not much new research has been conducted on the ingredient combo since then.

SAFETY AND TOLERANCE CONCERNS

- The ingredients in FDgard are generally recognized as safe by the Food and Drug Administration.

- The most common adverse effect associated with peppermint oil supplements is heartburn. This is because the oil relaxes smooth muscles throughout the digestive tract, potentially including the one separating your stomach and esophagus.

- People allergic to caraway seed should not use FDgard.

DOSING

- The manufacturer recommends dosing of two capsules, twice a day or as needed. Do not exceed six capsules per day.

- FDgard should be taken at least thirty minutes before or thirty minutes after food, with water. Do not take FDgard at the same time as antacid medications or H2 blocker acid-reducing drugs (Zantac, Pepcid). FDgard should be taken an hour before these medications. It can be taken at the same time as a proton-pump inhibitor (PPI) medication, or any acid-reducing drug that ends with *-prazole.*

- Swallow capsules whole or mix contents with applesauce. Do not chew.

THE BOTTOM LINE?

- Worth a try. While the evidence is still pretty limited, it's certainly promising enough to merit giving FDgard a try given the safety of the ingredients it contains.

Fennel (Seeds, Tea): Foeniculum vulgare

WHAT IT IS

Fennel is a flowering plant species in the carrot family. It is a flavorful herb with an aniselike flavor that's been used for centuries in Europe and China to relieve various forms of gastrointestinal distress. If you've ever dined out at an Indian restaurant, you may have noticed colorful, candy-coated seeds in a bowl by the entrance; these are fennel seeds, traditionally chewed as an after-meal digestive aid.

WHAT MARKETERS CLAIM IT DOES

- Reduces abdominal pain and gas, particularly associated with irritable bowel syndrome (IBS).

- Has antispasmodic properties and is a carminative (helps expel gas or reduces its formation).

WHAT IT ACTUALLY DOES

- Fennel has only been studied as a digestive aid for adults in combination with other herbal ingredients, like peppermint, ginger, curcumin, and licorice. There is limited to no evidence on the support of fennel seeds or fennel tea in relieving flatulence and IBS symptoms. Most of the support from fennel comes from anecdotal evidence.

- Isolated fennel seed oil or teas made from fennel seed have been studied in isolation to a limited degree in infants with colic, where they have shown promise as a natural remedy for symptoms.

SAFETY AND TOLERANCE CONCERNS

- Fennel seeds and teas derived from them are considered very safe for adults using them occasionally and in moderation to manage digestive complaints.

- Toxicologists have recently investigated fennel teas due to concerns about their levels of a natural compound called *estragole,* which may be carcinogenic (cancer causing) at higher doses. They were particularly concerned with instant fennel teas marketed as a colic remedy for infants, raising concerns that estragole concentrations may be inappropriately high for their low body weights.

DOSING

- There is no standard dose recommendation available for potential digestive benefits.

THE BOTTOM LINE?

- Worth a try for bloating that originates in the stomach and is accompanied by belching or gas pain, like from functional dyspepsia, classic indigestion, or aerophagia. At the end of the day, it's a nice warm cup of tea, so even if the fennel itself doesn't alleviate your bloating, the relaxing effect of a tea break may.

- To be on the safe side, don't share it with your colicky infants.

Florastor (Probiotic): Saccharomyces boulardii lyo CNCM I-745

WHAT IT IS

Florastor is a yeast-based probiotic supplement containing *Saccharomyces boulardii* Iyo CNCM I-745, a species/strain of yeast naturally found on the skins of certain tropical fruits. It is one of the oldest commercialized probiotic products and is the single-most researched one.

Unlike most commercial probiotic products, Florastor contains yeast, not bacteria. This means that Florastor is not killed by antibiotic medications.

WHAT MARKETERS CLAIM IT DOES

- Strengthens your digestive balance.

- Increases your body's production of lactase enzyme, improving lactose tolerance.

WHAT IT ACTUALLY DOES

- There is relatively strong evidence in support of Florastor's benefit in reducing diarrhea among people with irritable bowel syndrome (IBS) and preventing both traveler's diarrhea and antibiotic-associated diarrhea (AAD) in adults and children.

- Florastor may also be protective against opportunistic infections from *Clostridium difficile* (*C. diff*) when using antibiotics.

- Evidence to support the claim that Florastor improves lactose tolerance is much, much weaker. The claim is based on one tiny study conducted in 1986 that included only seven people. While it showed that Florastor taken four times daily substantially increased their production of lactase enzyme, it did not actually test whether they became less symptomatic when consuming dairy foods.

SAFETY AND TOLERANCE CONCERNS

- Florastor has a sixty-year track record of safety. Like all probiotics, it is safe for adults and children who are not immunocompromised.

- Each adult capsule contains about ⅓ gram of lactose. This minute dose should probably not pose a tolerance problem for lactose-intolerant people.

- Because Florastor contains yeast and not bacteria, it cannot contribute to risk of SIBO. For this reason, it is my probiotic of choice for patients undergoing antibiotic treatment to eradicate SIBO or who have a history of SIBO.

- The yeast in Florastor is an entirely different species from the one that causes vaginal yeast infections and oral thrush (*Candida albicans*). Therefore, Florastor cannot contribute to risk of candida infections.

DOSING

- Two capsules, one to two times daily.

- Since probiotic supplements do not colonize the colon permanently, any benefits you experience will stop within about a week of stopping use.

THE BOTTOM LINE?

- Worth a try for people with SIBO or a past history of SIBO who wish to use a probiotic when using antibiotics (or beyond).

- Skip it if you're lactose intolerant looking for a magic bullet to become more lactose tolerant. See entry on lactase enzyme for a better option.

Garlic Extract

SEE ENTRY

- Allicin

Ginger: Zingiber officinale

ALSO MARKETED AS

- Gingerol, Ginger Root, Ginger Root Extract, Ginger Tea

WHAT IT IS

Ginger is the root of an herbal plant that is native to Asia and has been used both as a culinary spice and for traditional medicinal purposes. It can be found as the whole root, ground into a powder, or dried in teas. The primary active compound in ginger is called *gingerol*.

WHAT MARKETERS CLAIM IT DOES

- Alleviates nausea.
- Soothes upset stomach.
- "Digestive support" aid.

WHAT IT ACTUALLY DOES

- There has been a lot of research assessing the effectiveness of ginger as an antiemetic (anti-nausea/vomiting) medication. The most encouraging evidence of benefit appears to be as a remedy for nausea in pregnancy, from chemotherapy, and in postoperative nausea and vomiting.
- Gingerol may also have a natural antispasmodic and muscle-relaxing effect, similar to that of peppermint oil, which can be helpful for abdominal pain.

SAFETY AND TOLERANCE CONCERNS

- Ginger extract may have blood-thinning properties, so you should not take it with blood-thinning medications (warfarin/Coumadin), aspirin, or in combination with supplements like gingko, vitamin E, or high-dose fish oil. Ginger might increase the risk of bleeding problems if you are taking one of these medications.
- Because of ginger's muscle-relaxing effect, ginger teas or supplements that break down in the stomach could cause heartburn in some people.

DOSING

- One gram of whole ginger root appears to be an effective dose for anti-nausea benefits.
- However, there is no standardization with ginger supplements, as some products include the whole herb and others just contain gingerol extract. Ginger teas and ginger chews are also available, and their gingerol content is undeclared.

- Worth a try for bloating that results from functional dyspepsia and for nausea that accompanies any type of bloating.

- A ginger tea or ginger chew may be a better form than a coated pill for bloating that originates in the stomach, as it enables maximum contact of the gingerol with the muscles of the stomach, but it may require experimentation to see which form, if any, is helpful for you.

L-glutamine

WHAT IT IS

L-glutamine is an amino acid, or one of the many building blocks of protein. It is considered a nonessential amino acid, meaning the body can make its own supply without having to obtain any directly from the diet. Protein-rich foods, such as meat, fish, beans, and dairy products, are high in glutamine. Glutamine happens to be a preferred source of energy for the cells that line the intestines, called *enterocytes*. L-glutamine is sold in powdered or pill forms.

WHAT MARKETERS CLAIM IT DOES

- Supports the lining and the healthy functioning of the gastrointestinal tract.

- Promotes digestive health.

- L-glutamine is a popular supplement recommended by alternative medicine practitioners for the purpose of "healing the gut" from inflammatory conditions. Among practitioners who believe in leaky gut syndrome, L-glutamine is commonly recommended based on a belief that it reduces intestinal permeability (leakiness) or improves gut barrier function.

WHAT IT ACTUALLY DOES

- Most scientific research into L-glutamine's effect on the gut relates to people with an inflammatory bowel condition called *Crohn's disease,* where it was shown to have no benefit in helping achieve remission even at very high levels of 30 grams.

- The notion that L-glutamine may help improve your gut's barrier function comes from research into critically ill, hospitalized patients under significant medical stress receiving intravenous (IV) nutrition. There is evidence suggesting that adding L-glutamine to the IV fluid bags may improve gut barrier function in patients recovering from major surgery, severe burns, or other medical traumas. The evidence, however, is not sufficient to have merited recommendations of routine use of IV glutamine supplementation in critically ill patients by the medical community.

- L-glutamine given by mouth as a pill or fed directly into the gut through liquid formulas has been tested and has generally shown no such benefit on gut barrier function in these critically ill patients.

- It has not been studied as an oral supplement in healthy people with other digestive issues, like bloating, SIBO, or irritable bowel syndrome (IBS). There is no evidence whatsoever that it helps improve food allergies or any adverse food reactions (sensitivities or intolerances).

SAFETY AND TOLERANCE CONCERNS

- Because L-glutamine is really just a protein, it's quite safe even at high doses of several grams per day for people whose kidneys function normally. You probably get 1–6 grams per day from your diet alone.

- If you are sensitive to the effects of monosodium glutamate (MSG), be careful with supplementing glutamine, as excess amounts can be converted into glutamate and provoke a response similar to that of MSG.

DOSING

- Oral supplement doses vary widely, from 500 milligrams (½ gram) to 5,000 milligrams (5 grams) and even higher. There is no standardization. Much of the research into oral L-glutamine (which showed no benefit for various conditions) used doses of about 7 grams (7,000 milligrams) per day.

THE BOTTOM LINE?

- Skip it. While L-glutamine is perfectly safe when taken by mouth, it's probably useless for bloating, SIBO, carbohydrate (or other food) intolerance, inflammatory bowel diseases, or general digestive function.

- Avoid L-glutamine infused directly into your veins at so-called infusion centers. This is not a regulated therapy and has not been shown to be beneficial for healthy people with digestive problems. Delivering any nutrients directly into your veins carries significant risks of infection, and these risks outweigh any demonstrated or theoretical benefits.

Glycerin Suppositories: Glycerol suppository

WHAT IT IS

Rectal suppositories are waxy, bullet-shaped medicines that you insert directly into your rectum, where they begin melting at your body's regular temperature. Glycerin is essentially vegetable oil.

Suppository laxatives are a pretty old-fashioned approach to managing constipation, and virtually all studies on glycerin suppositories were conducted in the 1950s and 1960s. Back in the day, they were typically compounded by pharmacists and sold over the counter as a constipation remedy. Nowadays, they're used regularly in hospitalized patients or minimally active elderly people in long-term-care facilities to prevent stool from becoming very dried out and impacted.

WHAT MARKETERS CLAIM IT DOES

- Provides rapid relief from constipation, promoting a bowel movement within minutes.

WHAT IT ACTUALLY DOES

- Glycerin has an osmotic effect, drawing water into the bowel in a manner that stimulates contractions and promotes bowel movements. It can soften bits of stool that are dried out and blocking the rectum as well. Often, the presence of a foreign object in the rectum can also stimulate the nerves, cause contractions, and promote evacuation of stool.

- No scientists have bothered researching these products in healthy adult populations for over fifty years except when comparing them to enemas as a way to clean out the colon before sigmoidoscopy procedures. (Enemas proved to be superior.)

- Most current research into the use of glycerin suppositories pertains to premature infants who are hospitalized, where they are being studied as a potential therapy to prevent feeding intolerance by stimulating intestinal motility. (So far, they don't seem to be helpful.)

- Given the lack of recent research, it's difficult to say whether glycerin suppositories are especially effective (or superior to other, more modern options) to address any of the various types of constipation that lead to bloating.

SAFETY AND TOLERANCE CONCERNS

- Regular usage may cause irritation of the delicate skin in your rectum. If you have an anal fissure, you should not use glycerin suppositories, as they will be irritating.

- Some people find that the osmotic (water-attracting) effect of glycerin can cause abdominal discomfort or cramps.

- Severe side effects may accompany overuse and include severe stomach/abdominal pain, blood in the stools, rectal bleeding, persistent urge to have a bowel movement, and/or persistent diarrhea.

DOSING

- Typical products are 2 grams of glycerin per suppository.

THE BOTTOM LINE?

- Worth a try for constipation resulting from severely delayed colon motility (colonic inertia) or pelvic floor dysfunction—for occasional use—ideally after all other laxative options have been exhausted. Water or mineral-oil enemas are far likelier to be effective—and less irritating to the skin—for regular use in these scenarios.

ALSO MARKETED AS

- STW 5

WHAT IT IS

Iberogast is a brand name of a liquid supplement that contains nine herbal extracts, including bitter candytuft, angelica, chamomile, caraway, St. Mary's thistle, lemon balm, peppermint, greater celandine, and licorice.

It was developed in Germany decades ago to address symptoms associated with functional dyspepsia, but here in the United States, it is marketed as a remedy for symptoms of irritable bowel syndrome (IBS).

WHAT MARKETERS CLAIM IT DOES

- Relieves symptoms associated with IBS and functional dyspepsia, such as stomach pain, abdominal cramps, bloating, gas, nausea, heartburn, diarrhea, and constipation.

WHAT IT ACTUALLY DOES

- There have been four clinical studies investigating Iberogast as a remedy for the symptoms of functional dyspepsia (chapter 5); three of them showed it to improve gastrointestinal symptoms better than a placebo treatment.

- While research into Iberogast's utility in IBS is limited, the available data are promising about whether it helps reduce abdominal pain and other IBS symptoms better than a placebo.

- To the extent that Iberogast may be helpful to some, it is not clear which of the product's nine herbal extracts are responsible for that benefit, as most of them have not been well studied individually.

SAFETY AND TOLERANCE CONCERNS

- While no adverse effects have been reported in the handful of small studies investigating Iberogast, the nature of the formulation—which contains extracts from nine distinct herbs—could pose risks of possible side effects. Of greatest concern may be the licorice extract.

- Pregnant women should avoid all products containing licorice, including Iberogast, due to risk of preterm labor.

- If you use diuretic medications that reduce potassium levels, licorice-containing supplements may cause a very serious drop in potassium levels. Examples of such drugs include Lasix (furosemide), Demadex (torsemide), Bumex (bumetanide), Edecrin (ethacrynic acid), Diuril (chlorothiazide), Microzide (hydrochlorothiazide), chlorthalidone, Indapamide, or metolazone. Do not take licorice-containing supplements if you use these medications.

- According to the manufacturer's brochure for health-care professionals, Iberogast contains the equivalent 33.33 milligrams of licorice root per milliliter, or 99.99 milligrams of licorice root for the three daily recommended doses. European safety guidelines suggest that up to 100 milligrams per day should be a safe dose of whole licorice root. In other words, if you don't exceed the recommended daily intake of Iberogast and you don't use medications that might interact with licorice root, it should be safe.

DOSING

- The recommended dose is twenty drops (1 milliliter) in water three times daily.

THE BOTTOM LINE?

- Worth a try for bloating from functional dyspepsia if you are not pregnant or using any potassium-depleting medications. Do not exceed the daily recommended dose.

Insoluble-Fiber Supplements

ALSO MARKETED AS

- FiberCon (Calcium Polycarbophil), Ground Flaxseed/Linseed, Linaza

WHAT IT IS

Insoluble-fiber supplements contain specific types of fiber that are able to absorb water in the gut and swell to create softer, bulkier stools. Insoluble fiber does not dissolve in water in the same way as soluble fiber does, so it does not form a gooey gel. Instead, it creates a bulky stool that stimulates the colon to contract and speeds up the transit time of stool passing through a sluggish gut. Insoluble fiber can be derived from various natural sources or synthesized in a lab.

Wheat bran and hempseeds are also insoluble fiber–rich dietary supplements, but it's unclear whether they are able to hold as much water as flaxseeds and calcium polycarbophil.

WHAT MARKETERS CLAIM IT DOES

- Relieves constipation.

WHAT IT ACTUALLY DOES

- Various forms of insoluble fiber, including the main ingredient in FiberCon (calcium polycarbophil) and ground flaxseeds, have been well studied in constipated populations and shown to be of benefit.

- Specifically, these bulk-forming fiber supplements improve stool frequency (pooping more often) in people who are constipated for a variety of reasons, whether due to old age, irritable bowel syndrome (IBS), or even nervous system diseases or injuries that affect their bowel function.

- The type of fiber in FiberCon also seems to improve stool form, making things easier to pass, and can reduce abdominal pain associated with the urge to defecate.

- Research suggests that ground flaxseeds (also called *linseeds,* or *linaza*) may be a more effective constipation remedy than whole flaxseeds.

SAFETY AND TOLERANCE CONCERNS

- Fiber supplements are safe for anyone without swallowing problems. Be sure to take fiber supplements with the recommended amount of water listed on package labels.

- Do not take any fiber supplement if you think your stool may be impacted, which means it is blocking your colon due to a hard mass of dried-out stool. A good rule of thumb: If you haven't moved your bowels in five to seven days, it's best to avoid fiber supplements unless a doctor gives you the green light.

- Some forms of insoluble fiber, such as wheat bran, are likely to make diarrhea worse. If you have diarrhea, see entry on soluble-fiber supplements for more suitable options.

- Certain fiber supplements also contain added fiber from inulin, chicory root, yacon, or other prebiotic ingredients, like fructo-oligosaccharides. Read all ingredient labels and avoid products with these ingredients. They will likely be gassy and worsen your bloating if you are backed up.

DOSING

The effective dose of insoluble fiber depends on the source. For example:

- FiberCon: two pills once daily (1 gram). You may take a second dose if needed, but do not exceed four pills per day. Take with at least 8 ounces of water per serving.

- Ground flaxseed/flaxseed meal: 2 tablespoons powder (3 grams).

- You can mix flaxseed meal into oatmeal, smoothies, cereals, yogurts, or liquids.

THE BOTTOM LINE?

- Worth a try for constipation from IBS, slow transit, opioid medications, or a low-fiber diet.

Lactase Enzyme

ALSO MARKETED AS

- Lactaid Dietary Supplements; DairyAssist; Dairy Aid

WHAT IT IS

Lactase is a human digestive enzyme produced by cells in the small intestine. It breaks down the natural milk sugar, lactose, into its two component parts during digestion so that they can be absorbed. Some individuals do not produce sufficient amounts of lactase after childhood and therefore may not be able to absorb lactose from the dairy foods in their diet. This is called *lactose intolerance,* and it results in intestinal gas (farting), abdominal bloating and pain, diarrhea, and/or nausea after consuming foods with lactose.

Lactase enzyme supplements enable lactose-intolerant people to break down lactose in their small intestines so that it can be absorbed, preventing the symptoms associated with lactose intolerance.

WHAT MARKETERS CLAIM IT DOES

- Reduces or prevents gas, bloating, nausea, and diarrhea when taken along with a lactose-containing dairy food.

WHAT IT ACTUALLY DOES

- When taken in a sufficient dose right as you begin to eat dairy foods, lactase enzyme does what the marketers say it does.

- Several studies have investigated and confirmed the effectiveness of lactase supplements in both capsule and tablet form.

- Lactase enzymes can also be added to milk, and this is how marketers make liquid cow's milk and products made from it (yogurts, ice cream, cottage cheese, cream cheese, kefir) lactose-free.

SAFETY AND TOLERANCE CONCERNS

- Lactase enzyme supplements have been well tested for safety. There are really no risks or contraindications for their use.

- Some lactase enzyme supplement products are formulated with an inactive ingredient called *mannitol.* Mannitol itself is an indigestible, fermentable carbohydrate and can cause gas in people sensitive to the polyol FODMAP family. Look for products that do not contain this filler ingredient if available.

DOSING

- Lactase units are measured in ALU, or *acid lactase units.* This refers to how much lactose the enzyme can break down in a certain period of time. When using lactase supplements, it's important to consume enough of the active ingredient to cover the amount of lactose in your meal. You must also take the supplement along with the first bite of your dairy-containing meal or snack; it doesn't work when taken after you finish eating.

- 3,000 ALU can help digest about 20 grams of lactose from milk (~1.5 cups), but 6,000 ALU provides a greater benefit.

- For digesting larger amounts of lactose (50 grams, equivalent to 4 cups of milk), 10,000 ALU has shown benefits in symptom reduction.

- Most products on the market recommend a dose of 9,000 ALU per meal, which should be sufficient for most dairy-containing meals.

- If you are relying on a broad-spectrum digestive enzyme supplement to help you digest dairy foods, you should check the amount contained in the product to make sure it contains 6,000–9,000 ALU of lactase.

- Worth a try. If you're lactose intolerant and don't want to give up high-lactose dairy foods, lactase enzyme supplements may help you be able to have your cheesecake . . . and eat it too.

Magnesium: Mg

WHAT IT IS

Magnesium is an essential mineral that is present in the body and is considered an electrolyte. It plays a key role in many important processes, including regulating nerve and muscle function; regulating blood sugar levels and blood pressure; bone building; and synthesizing proteins and DNA. The recommended dietary allowance for magnesium depends on age, sex, and pregnancy status, but for nonpregnant adults over eighteen years of age, the recommended intake is 310 milligrams to 420 milligrams per day.

Magnesium is naturally present in many foods. The richest dietary sources include nuts, seeds, cocoa powder, broccoli, beets, asparagus, peas, bananas, oatmeal, whole wheat/wheat bran, and milk. Magnesium supplements come in different forms, such as magnesium oxide, sulfate, and citrate. High-dose magnesium oxide is marketed as an over-the-counter drug (e.g., Phillips' Milk of Magnesia).

WHAT MARKETERS CLAIM IT DOES

- Has a laxative effect.

WHAT IT ACTUALLY DOES

- When taken as a supplement in doses greater than 350 milligrams, magnesium has a laxative effect. The excess, unabsorbed magnesium salts draw water into the bowel through osmosis and stimulate intestinal motility. If you've ever had to clean out your bowels in preparation for a colonoscopy, you may have been prescribed a very high dose of magnesium citrate to do the trick.

- Studies have suggested that magnesium may be superior to other supplements, such as bulk (fiber) laxatives or sorbitol, in producing more bowel movements and more normal stool consistency among constipated people.

SAFETY AND TOLERANCE CONCERNS

- The primary side effect of high-dose magnesium is diarrhea. Stomachaches and nausea are also a possibility.

- Because magnesium must be processed by the kidneys, people with impaired kidney function should not use high-dose magnesium, either as a laxative or an antacid. Doing so may increase the risk of magnesium toxicity. Somewhat high doses of magnesium should not pose a health risk in people with well-functioning kidneys because they eliminate excess magnesium in the urine.

- Extremely high doses of magnesium-containing laxatives and antacids (>5,000 milligrams per day) have been associated with magnesium toxicity. Magnesium toxicity presents as nausea, vomiting, facial flushing, low blood pressure, urine retention, depression, lethargy before progressing to muscle weakness, difficulty breathing, and/or irregular heartbeats.

- Magnesium can interfere with several medications.

- Separate magnesium-rich supplements or medications from oral bisphosphonate drugs (Fosamax, Actonel) by at least two hours.

- People on antibiotics or diuretics should speak with their doctor before using magnesium supplements.

DOSING

- For constipation, start with 400 milligrams at night. If it does not produce an adequate laxative response the next morning, increase your dose to 600 milligrams. You may increase by 200 milligrams per night until you reach 1,000 milligrams. Do not split the dose into separate sittings; magnesium works best when the full dose is delivered all at once.

- In my experience, if 1,000 milligrams of magnesium does not produce an adequate laxative effect, then you should consider layering on a different type of laxative or switching approaches entirely; taking more is not likely to help. See entries under senna, N-acetyl cysteine (NAC), and insoluble-fiber supplements for complementary supplement options. See chapter 7 on constipation for over-the-counter and prescription medication options as well.

- All forms of magnesium—citrate, sulfate, malate, fumarate, oxide, hydroxide—should be beneficial. No need to spend more for chelated magnesium; the cheaper stuff works just as well.

- Phillips' Milk of Magnesia is a brand-name magnesium-based laxative sold as an over-the-counter medication and contains 1,200 milligrams of magnesium per tablespoon of liquid and 500 milligrams per caplet.

THE BOTTOM LINE?

- Worth a try. Magnesium is one of the most effective remedies for constipation I employ in my clinical practice for patients with slow-transit constipation, irritable bowel syndrome (IBS), and opioid-induced constipation. It will be less effective if your constipation is caused by pelvic floor dysfunction, but is still worth a try.

N-Acetyl Cysteine

ALSO MARKETED AS

- NAC, Acetyl Cysteine

N-acetyl cysteine (NAC) is a modified form of the amino acid, or protein building block, L-cysteine. In the body, NAC is converted into a powerful antioxidant called *glutathione;* taking it as a supplement has been shown to increase levels of this antioxidant. NAC is not an essential nutrient, and there is no recommended daily allowance.

WHAT MARKETERS CLAIM IT DOES

- Enhance liver's detoxifying function.
- Liver support.

WHAT IT ACTUALLY DOES

- NAC has two well-studied benefits: It may help improve lung function in people with chronic obstructive pulmonary disease (COPD), and it is used to counteract acetaminophen (Tylenol) poisoning/overdose.

- NAC's benefit for COPD has to do with its ability to thin out mucus (and other sticky stuff); it does this by breaking down a specific type of chemical bond. This action of NAC also has effects in the gut and may be responsible for a lesser-known benefit that has not yet been studied by researchers: NAC supplements work as a laxative. NAC makes it easier for a slow colon to propel a sticky poo by making it less viscous. (This is the same reason it makes it easier for diseased lungs to propel sticky mucus out.)

- While NAC is also used as a detoxifying agent of sorts, it is probably not in the way that many people envision. Rather, NAC is used to counteract acetaminophen (Tylenol) poisoning. It works by replenishing the antioxidant glutathione in the liver, which is depleted by the acetaminophen overdose.

SAFETY AND TOLERANCE CONCERNS

- Because NAC is essentially a protein building block, it is very safe.
- Some people may experience headache or gastrointestinal symptoms at very high doses of 1,200 milligrams twice daily.
- NAC should not be taken with the heart medication nitroglycerine without supervision from a physician, as it can cause unsafe lowering of blood pressure.

DOSING

- In our practice, we find that 600 milligrams of NAC taken twice daily can be very helpful as a laxative, particularly in our patients who have not responded adequately to magnesium supplements.

- Because NAC works via a different mechanism than magnesium, the two supplements can be used together in a complementary fashion as laxatives for people with stubborner cases of constipation. (See entry on magnesium for details.)

THE BOTTOM LINE?

- Worth a try for constipation of all causes.

Oregano Oil: Origanum vulgare

WHAT IT IS

Oregano is a common food herb that is indigenous to Mediterranean countries.

WHAT MARKETERS CLAIM IT DOES

- Alternative medicine practitioners claim it is an herbal antibiotic that can kill harmful bacteria in the gut (and treat SIBO) in lieu of prescription medications. They also claim it is an antifungal that can treat fungal infections, including candida infections that reside in the digestive tract.

- Because it is illegal for supplement marketers to make "drug" claims that their products can treat or cure any disease, package labels generally do not carry any such promises.

WHAT IT ACTUALLY DOES

- Oregano oil does have toxic and inhibitory effects against certain fungi and bacteria on plants and in test tubes, likely as the result of a compound called *carvacrol*. But just because a compound can kill microorganisms in a test tube (or on a plant or on the surface of a food product), that does not mean it has comparable effects inside the human body.

- There have been no controlled human studies investigating any antibiotic or antifungal effects of oregano oil. Therefore, it is not clear what—if anything—oregano oil does in the human digestive tract.

SAFETY AND TOLERANCE CONCERNS

- There appear to be no safety risks associated with the use of oregano oil products so long as you are not allergic to oregano.

- People with a salicylate allergy/intolerance should not use oregano oil.

DOSING

- No dose has been established for use of oregano oil in treating GI symptoms due to lack of any scientific research on the topic.

THE BOTTOM LINE?

- Skip it. While it's most likely to be safe and well tolerated, oregano oil is not an antibiotic or an antifungal and should not be taken as such.

- There is no scientific evidence that oregano oil effectively treats SIBO on its own or in combination with other herbal products.

- Pancrelipase

WHAT IT IS

Pancreatin is an enzyme supplement that mirrors the digestive enzyme trio normally secreted by the human pancreas. It combines three enzymes: amylase (for digesting starch), protease (for digesting protein), and lipase (for digesting fat). Some products may also include trypsin and chymotrypsin, other enzymes from the pancreas that help digest proteins.

It may be animal-derived (usually from pigs) or vegetarian, usually from a type of mold called *Aspergillus*.

This product differs from broad-spectrum digestive enzyme products in that the doses of amylase, protease, and lipase may be higher. It does not contain other types of enzymes to help digest sugars and fiber.

The dietary supplement pancreatin is an unregulated version of prescription digestive enzymes known as *pancreatic enzyme replacement therapy* (*PERT*) used by people whose bodies do not secrete enough pancreatic enzymes (cystic fibrosis or pancreatic insufficiency.) The main differences are:

- The supplement pancreatin is generally formulated with much lower doses of lipase than the prescription version. However, a few high-potency products do have lipase levels in the same range as prescription products on the lower end of the scale.

- The supplement version is not well regulated, so products may not have standardized doses; they can vary from batch to batch or have higher or lower doses than those listed on the label.

- The supplement version may or may not be *enteric coated,* or coated with an acid-resistant capsule so that the enzymes survive intact until reaching the small intestine.

WHAT MARKETERS CLAIM IT DOES

- Supports digestion.
- Improves/promotes nutrient absorption.
- Prevents occasional symptoms of indigestion.

WHAT IT ACTUALLY DOES

- Two very small, randomized controlled trials have examined the effects of giving healthy people lipase before a high-fat meal. Those who took the lipase reported feeling less bloating, gas, fullness, and nausea after eating compared to those who were given a placebo. The lipase doses used in these studies were much, much higher than those contained in a standard pancreatin dietary supplement.

- One small study showed no benefit of prescription pancreatic enzymes on symptoms in people with functional dyspepsia (chapter 5) compared to a placebo.

- Various protein- and starch-digesting enzymes have not shown much of a benefit on digestive symptoms in people without pancreatic insufficiency, though in fairness, they've barely been examined at all.

SAFETY AND TOLERANCE CONCERNS

- Digestive enzymes should generally be quite safe.

- One hypothetical safety issue with digestive enzyme cocktails pertains to excessive exposure to lipase, which can damage the colon. Very high doses of supplemental lipase can cause a scarlike thickening of the colon's walls that leads to constipation and possibly even obstructions, though admittedly, this should not be a risk with the relatively low levels of lipase contained in the dietary supplement products I've reviewed.

- On a separate note, some brands of digestive enzyme products contain prebiotic ingredients like fructo-oligosaccharides (FOS) or inulin (chicory root fiber) that may cause gas and bloating in people already predisposed to bloating.

DOSING

- Dosing is not at all standardized. It may be listed in milligrams or grams of pancreatin, or in units (USP) of each component enzyme, or both.

- There are no dosing guidelines for healthy people who do not have a deficiency of pancreatic enzymes.

THE BOTTOM LINE?

- Skip it. Most bloating that results from malabsorption is triggered by unabsorbed sugars like lactose or fructose, or various plant fibers. The ingredients in pancreatin will not help you digest these dietary compounds.

- If you actually have a medical condition called *pancreatic insufficiency,* it should be treated under the supervision of a doctor with a standardized enzyme product that has higher levels of lipase and whose enteric coating has been tested and shown to be effective.

- If you experience chronic bloating and diarrhea following the removal of your gallbladder, it may be a sign of bile acid diarrhea. This is usually treated with medications called *bile acid sequestrants,* not with pancreatic enzyme supplements. Talk to your doctor.

Papain: Carica papaya

ALSO MARKETED AS

- Papaya Enzyme

WHAT IT IS

Papain is a protein-digesting enzyme extracted from the fruit of a papaya tree. It is not the same enzyme manufactured by the human body to digest proteins.

WHAT MARKETERS CLAIM IT DOES

- "Natural digestive enzyme support."

- Promotes nutrient absorption.

WHAT IT ACTUALLY DOES

- Papain has not been studied for a potential role as a human digestive aid. It is therefore not clear what effect, if any, papain has on digestive symptoms or nutrient absorption.

SAFETY AND TOLERANCE CONCERNS

- People with an allergy to papaya should not take papain.

- Papain may have a mild blood-thinning effect, so you should not take it with blood-thinning medications (warfarin/Coumadin), aspirin, or in combination with supplements like gingko, vitamin E, or high-dose fish oil.

DOSING

- 2.4 million FCC papain units (PU) is the maximum dose per serving one should consume in a sitting according to guidelines by Health Canada. (The U.S. government does not issue guidelines.)

THE BOTTOM LINE?

- Skip it.

- It's not likely to help your bloating, though it's also not likely to hurt you so long as you don't take any of the medications listed above that might interact with it.

- I personally don't recommend it to my patients, based on the lack of evidence and the fact that protease (protein-digesting enzyme) deficiency isn't likely a bloated person's problem; if it were, then they'd need a more standardized preparation of animal-derived pancreatic enzyme replacement therapy anyway (see chapter 13).

Peppermint Oil Capsules: Mentha piperita

ALSO MARKETED AS

- Pepogest, IBgard, Heather's Tummy Tamers

Peppermint is a wild herb widely used in beverages, teas, and as a flavoring/scent in many products. Peppermint oil supplement capsules are *not* the same thing as peppermint essential oil and should not be confused. Essential oils can be harmful when taken by mouth in excess doses.

WHAT MARKETERS CLAIM IT DOES

- Helps reduce bowel discomfort.

- Helps reduce abdominal pain and cramping, particularly among people with irritable bowel syndrome (IBS).

- May help reduce bowel urgency in IBS.

WHAT IT ACTUALLY DOES

- Peppermint oil has a natural antispasmodic and smooth muscle–relaxing effect.

- Peppermint oil in enteric-coated capsules—or pills with an acid-resistant coating designed to survive the stomach and break down in the gut—has been pretty well studied in people with IBS. It is one of the remedies with the best evidence in support of its helpfulness, mainly related to reducing abdominal pain and cramping, compared to placebo pills.

- Peppermint oil appears to be more effective and potent in its antispasmodic effects than peppermint tea due to a higher concentration of active ingredients and the delivery of ingredients directly to the gut rather than to the stomach.

- There is much less research into the effect of peppermint oil as a remedy for upper-abdominal bloating and discomfort resulting from functional dyspepsia (chapter 5). A few small studies that tested peppermint oil in combination with caraway oil have shown promise, though it's unclear whether it was the peppermint oil, the caraway oil, or the combination of both that was responsible for the results.

SAFETY AND TOLERANCE CONCERNS

- The most common adverse effect associated with peppermint oil supplements is heartburn. This is because the oil relaxes smooth muscles throughout the digestive tract, including the one separating your stomach and esophagus. Choosing a product with a high-quality enteric coating should help prevent this side effect.

- Peppermint oil may increase levels of the drug cyclosporine in the body. Consult a physician if you take this medication and plan to take peppermint oil.

- High intakes can also cause nausea, loss of appetite, heart problems, loss of balance, and other nervous system problems. Excessive doses of peppermint oil can be toxic, causing kidney failure.

- Studies have shown that between 0.2 and 0.4 milliliters of enteric-coated peppermint oil, taken three times daily, is an effective dose for alleviating abdominal pain among people with IBS. In my clinical practice, most patients get adequate symptom relief with one or two capsules per day.

- It can take several hours for enteric-coated peppermint oil capsules to reach its target location, so you should consider taking it at bedtime for relief of early-morning symptoms, or taking it in the morning for relief of post-lunch symptoms. Start with one dose per day to make sure you tolerate it before adding additional doses as needed.

THE BOTTOM LINE?

- Worth a try for bloating of any origin accompanied by lower-abdominal cramping or pain.

Prebiotic Supplements

WHAT THEY ARE

Prebiotics are plant-derived fibers known to resist digestion in the small intestine and reach the colon. They are highly fermentable by certain species of beneficial bacteria residing in the colon and are often referred to as the "food" for these probiotic bacteria. In order for a fiber to be considered prebiotic, it must selectively feed and nourish beneficial species of bacteria known to promote human health.

Prebiotics may be sold as a separate supplement or as an ingredient in various digestive enzyme, probiotic, or protein powder supplements under the names:

- Inulin

- Chicory root fiber/extract

- Resistant starch

- Jerusalem artichoke fiber/flour/extract

- Fructo-oligosaccharides (FOS)

- Oligofructose

- Yacon

WHAT MARKETERS CLAIM IT DOES

- Improves gut health.

- Promotes the growth of "good" colon bacteria.

- Reduces gut permeability.

- Reduces IBS symptoms, including constipation.
- Enhances calcium absorption.

WHAT IT ACTUALLY DOES

- Prebiotic-rich foods and dietary supplements have been shown to have a variety of health benefits.

    Prebiotics increase populations of certain favorable bacterial species in the gut—namely, those in the *Bifidobacteria* and *Lactobacilli* genera. (In fact, prebiotic supplements may do a better job of this than taking probiotic pills loaded with these actual bacteria!)

    The increased populations of *Bifidobacteria* and *Lactobacilli* result in increased production of the metabolic by-products they produce called *short-chain fatty acids* (*SCFAs*). SCFAs have been credited with a variety of health benefits. They feed the cells of your intestines, ensuring that the protective mucous barrier in your gut remains strong and intact. They also acidify the colon slightly, which prevents certain metabolic processes known to promote colon cancer risk.

    Prebiotic fiber has been shown to improve calcium absorption from the diet.

    Inulin supplementation is being investigated for its potential benefit in people with type 2 diabetes and other metabolic diseases. There is promising evidence suggesting it may help with blood sugar control.

- While randomized controlled trials in healthy, constipated people without IBS suggest that inulin may be helpful in softening and increasing frequency of stools, there is almost no scientific evidence to support the use of prebiotics for people with IBS. Studies thus far have not shown an improvement in abdominal pain and bloating with inulin use.

SAFETY AND TOLERANCE CONCERNS

- Prebiotic supplements are just a form of fiber. They are very safe.

- Despite the many objective health-promoting benefits of prebiotic foods and supplements, however, they can contribute to *substantial* gas and bloating in susceptible individuals. This is particularly the case for people whose bloating originates in the gut.

- Tolerance in healthy people *without IBS* suggested that mild symptoms of gas, bloating, and flatulence kicked in at doses of 5–8 grams of prebiotics.

- Scientific studies of prebiotic tolerance in people with IBS are lacking. In our clinical practice, however, we've observed that doses of inulin as low as 0.5–1.0 grams can trigger gas pain and abdominal discomfort in patients with IBS. So if you've got IBS or are prone to bloating, tread carefully with any product you encounter that lists any prebiotic ingredients or claims.

DOSING

- Commercially available prebiotic supplements typically contain between 3 and 7 grams of combined prebiotics per recommended dose.

- By way of comparison, the average amount of prebiotics in a 3-ounce serving of common foods is as follows:

  Jerusalem artichoke: 18 grams inulin and 13 grams oligofructose

  Raw garlic: 12 grams inulin and 5 grams oligofructose

  Raw leek: 7 grams inulin and 5 grams oligofructose

  Raw onion: 4 grams inulin and 4 grams oligofructose

  Artichoke: 4 grams inulin and 0.5 grams oligofructose

  Wheat bran: 3 grams inulin and 3 grams oligofructose

  Boiled asparagus: 2 grams inulin and 2 grams oligofructose

THE BOTTOM LINE?

- Avoid if you have IBS or any bloating that originates in the intestines.

- If your bloating originates in the stomach and you tolerate the prebiotic-rich foods listed above, you could give prebiotic supplements a try if you wanted to support the health of your gut microbiota. But start with a very conservative dose. A little goes a long way!

Probiotic Supplements (Assorted Varieties)

WHAT IT IS

Probiotics are a broad category of supplements that contain microorganisms—bacteria or yeast—taken with the purpose of conferring a health benefit. Commercially available products may contain a single species/strain of organism or a cocktail of multiple different ones. When sold as a supplement, probiotics can be found in powder, liquid, tablet, or capsule forms.

As is the protocol for naming bacteria and fungi, probiotics are identified by the Latin names of their genus (the first, capitalized word or initial) and species (the second word). Some products will also identify a particular strain within the species, and this generally contains a combination of letters and/or numbers listed after the species.

Probiotic bacteria or yeasts may also be found naturally in cultured or fermented food/beverage products, such as yogurt, kefir, kimchi, kvass, sauerkraut, and kombucha.

WHAT MARKETERS CLAIM IT DOES

- Restore the balance between "good" and "bad" bacteria in the gut that can be disturbed by illness, antibiotic treatment, environmental factors, and diet.

- Support digestive regularity (regular bowel movements).

- Promote overall digestive system health.

- Promote immune health.

WHAT IT ACTUALLY DOES

- This depends entirely on what species/strain of probiotic you are taking and for what problem. Since the vast majority of commercially available probiotic products have *not* been tested in humans to verify that they have any effect on health, it is difficult to know whether a randomly chosen probiotic will be helpful for a particular problem you are looking to address.

- Probiotic supplements have not been shown to colonize the human gut permanently or measurably change/modify the human gut microbiota. Therefore, if you do experience any benefits from taking a probiotic supplement, these benefits will cease within about a week of stopping use.

- The best evidence of benefit from certain probiotic supplements pertains to managing traveler's diarrhea, diarrhea as a side effect from antibiotic use, and acute diarrhea from illness—particularly among children. The species with the best evidence of benefit for diarrhea include:

    Lactobacillus rhamnosus

    Lactobacillus rhamnosus GG (including Culturelle)

    Saccharomyces boulardii (including Florastor)

    Bifidobacterium lactis

    The evidence of probiotics benefiting people with irritable bowel syndrome (IBS) is weaker, but promising. Some evidence suggests that certain products may improve abdominal pain and help normalize stool patterns and consistency. The species that have shown the most potential thus far include:

    Bifidobacterium infantis (including Align)

    Bifidobacterium lactis

    Lactobacillus rhamnosus

    Lactobacillus rhamnosus GG (including Culturelle)

    Lactobacillus casei (e.g., Bio-K+)

    Lactobacillus acidophilus

    Lactobacillus reuteri

    Saccharomyces boulardii (including Florastor)

SAFETY AND TOLERANCE CONCERNS

- Probiotics are generally considered very safe for most everyone except sick infants and immunocompromised people.

- The one exception is among people with a history of SIBO (chapter 8), who are prone to overgrowing even "good" bacteria in their small intestines. Align and all other bacterial probiotics may "seed" the small bowel and induce a recurrence. Similarly, if you're at high risk for developing SIBO due to having low stomach acid levels from age, an autoimmune disease that decreases stomach acid levels, or use of an acid-reducing medication that ends with *-prazole,* taking bacterial probiotics may increase this risk.

DOSING

- In research studies, effective doses generally range from 5 billion to 40 billion CFUs per day, depending on the product and the condition being studied.

THE BOTTOM LINE?

- Worth a try if you choose a specific probiotic supplement that has a demonstrated benefit for the problem you are looking to solve. See entries under Align, Culturelle, Florastor, and VSL #3 for more details about these relatively well-researched products. Be aware that in general, probiotics are rarely a silver bullet for digestive issues; if they confer a benefit, it's likely to be a modest one.

- Skip bacterial probiotics if you have a history of SIBO (chapter 8) or are at high risk for developing SIBO. Yeast-based probiotics, such as those in the *Saccharomyces* genus, are safer. (See: Florastor.)

Senna

ALSO MARKETED AS

- Senokot, Smooth Move Tea

WHAT IT IS

Senna is a natural laxative derived from a plant in the legume family. It is marketed as a laxative in many forms, both as a dietary supplement and an over-the-counter drug. Its leaves or pods may be used to formulate a laxative tea, or its active compounds, called *sennosides,* can be extracted to form a capsule-based laxative. Senna is also available as an ingredient in rectal suppositories or enemas.

WHAT MARKETERS CLAIM IT DOES

- Gentle overnight relief of constipation.

WHAT IT ACTUALLY DOES

- Senna is well established as a stimulant laxative. It triggers contractions of the colon wall and increases secretions, both of which have the effect of speeding along stool and increasing its moisture content.

SAFETY AND TOLERANCE CONCERNS

- Like other stimulant laxatives, senna is probably more appropriate for occasional use than as a daily pillar of your bowel regimen. There are some concerns about the safety of stimulant laxatives like senna for daily, long-term use—particularly regarding the possibility that they can be dependency-forming.

- The most common side effects include abdominal cramping and/or diarrhea.

- People who use the medication digoxin should consult their doctor before using senna. Do not use senna while pregnant or nursing.

DOSING

- Take capsules or tea at bedtime to promote a bowel movement the following morning. Rectal suppositories should produce a bowel movement within an hour.

- For dietary supplements, capsules generally contain 8.6 milligrams of sennosides.

- For senna products marketed as over-the-counter laxative drugs, like Ex-Lax, the dose is stronger (15 milligrams of sennosides).

THE BOTTOM LINE?

- Worth a try for constipation of all origins if osmotic laxatives like magnesium, high-dose vitamin C, and/or MiraLAX don't get the job done.

Soluble-Fiber Supplements

ALSO MARKETED AS

- Citrucel, Benefiber, Psyllium Husk, Metamucil, Konsyl, Acacia Fiber, Heather's Tummy Fiber Regular Girl

WHAT IT IS

Soluble-fiber supplements are isolated fiber sources that dissolve in water to form a bulky, viscous (thick and gooey) gel in the gut. Soluble fiber slows down the transit time of stool passing through the gut, absorbing and retaining excess water so that stools become soft, formed, and cohesive. Soluble fiber can be isolated from various natural sources or synthesized in a lab.

Not all fiber supplements are pure or even predominantly soluble fiber, and so they will act differently in the gut. See the entry under insoluble-fiber supplements for a discussion of fiber products not listed on this page.

WHAT MARKETERS CLAIM IT DOES

- "Helps you stay regular."

- Relieves constipation.

WHAT IT ACTUALLY DOES

- Soluble fiber has a regulating effect on bowel function, helping to manage both diarrhea (by helping to slow down stools and improve their form) *and* constipation (by adding bulk to stools and helping them retain moisture).

- In reality, soluble fiber is probably more helpful in managing diarrhea than constipation. Some people with constipation—particularly opioid-induced constipation (OIC) or constipation from a low-fiber or grain-free/Paleo-style diet—will probably find soluble-fiber supplements helpful to improve their constipation and therefore alleviate their bloating.

SAFETY AND TOLERANCE CONCERNS

- Fiber supplements are extremely safe for anyone without swallowing problems. Be sure to take fiber supplements with the recommended amount of water listed on package labels.

- Do not take any fiber supplement if you think your stool may be impacted, which is a blockage of the intestine caused by a hard mass of dried-out stool. A good rule of thumb: If you haven't moved your bowels in five to seven days, it's best to avoid fiber supplements unless a doctor gives you the green light.

- People whose constipation results from irritable bowel syndrome (IBS-C), slow-transit constipation, or pelvic floor dysfunction may find soluble fiber uncomfortable and bloating in and of itself—like "cement" or a "brick" in the gut.

- Certain forms of soluble fiber are more fermentable (gassy) than others—particularly if they contain inulin, chicory root, yacon, or other prebiotic ingredients, like fructo-oligosaccharides. Read all ingredient labels, and avoid products with these ingredients.

- Psyllium husk fiber, the main ingredient in Konsyl and Metamucil, may be gassier than the type of fiber in Citrucel (methylcellulose) or Benefiber (wheat dextrin).

- If you have celiac disease, avoid fiber products derived from wheat, such as Benefiber. This product is, however, suitable for those on a low-FODMAP diet.

- Avoid fiber wafers, bars, and cereals. They will almost certainly contain very-high-FODMAP additives that will worsen gas and bloating.

DOSING

- A dose of 2 grams of soluble fiber is typically an effective dose, and it should be taken with 8 ounces of water. The amount of product you will need to use to achieve this dose will vary by brand. For example:

    Citrucel: 1 tablespoon powder or four pills

    Benefiber: 2 teaspoon powder

    Heather's Tummy Fiber (acacia): 1 teaspoon powder

Metamucil: 1 tablespoon regular-flavored powder or 1 teaspoon Metamucil-Free (unflavored) and sugar-free flavored powder, or five capsules

Konsyl: 1 teaspoon original powder or 2 teaspoons orange powder, or six psyllium capsules

THE BOTTOM LINE?

- Worth a try for bloating that results from opioid-induced constipation or a low-fiber diet.

- Also worth a try if you have irritable bowel syndrome that's diarrhea predominant (even if that's not what causes your bloating).

Vitamin C: Ascorbic acid

WHAT IT IS

Vitamin C is an essential nutrient for human health. It plays a key role in many important body processes, including wound healing, collagen production, helping cells create usable energy, and protecting cells from oxidative damage. The recommended dietary allowance for vitamin C is 75 milligrams per day for adult women and 90 milligrams per day for adult men.

Vitamin C is a water-soluble vitamin. That means excess amounts of it are filtered from the blood by the kidneys and excreted in the urine. Because of this, it is quite difficult (though not impossible) for a person to experience toxicity from oral doses of vitamin C, though high doses can increase your risk of developing kidney stones.

WHAT MARKETERS CLAIM IT DOES

- Supports the immune system.

- Helps absorb iron from supplements and food.

- Antioxidant.

WHAT IT ACTUALLY DOES

- While vitamin C supplements may have a variety of effects in the body, their main effect of interest for our purposes are that of a laxative when taken in very high doses.

- In doses greater than 2,000 milligrams, vitamin C acts as a laxative. This is because the body can only absorb a limited amount of vitamin C at a time, so excess amounts remain in the bowel and have an osmotic effect (draw water into the bowel) similar to that of magnesium. It will not contribute to intestinal gas.

- If you're constipated, this may help you move your bowels in a more normal way. If you're not constipated, this may give you diarrhea.

SAFETY AND TOLERANCE CONCERNS

- The main side effect or concern with high-dose vitamin C is diarrhea and/or indigestion.

- People with a personal or family history of kidney stones may not be good candidates for doses of vitamin C in excess of 1,000 milligrams/day, as it can increase risk of stone formation in susceptible people.

DOSING

- For a laxative effect, adults can take 2,000 milligrams (2 grams) of vitamin C in a single dose. This dose is considered the tolerable upper intake level (UL) established by the Institute of Medicine.

- Do not exceed this dose in a single day. Children should not take such high doses of vitamin C.

THE BOTTOM LINE?

- Worth a try for constipation that results from a variety of causes.

VSL #3

WHAT IT IS

VSL #3 is a probiotic supplement containing eight different species of bacteria, primarily from the *Bifidobacteria* and *Lactobacillus* genera. It contains a much higher dose of bacterial colony-forming units (CFUs) compared to other leading probiotic brands and comes in both over-the-counter and prescription strengths. It is sold refrigerated and must be dispensed by your pharmacist.

VSL #3 is among the best-studied commercial probiotics on the U.S. market.

WHAT MARKETERS CLAIM IT DOES

- "For the dietary management of irritable bowel syndrome, ulcerative colitis, and ileal pouch."

WHAT IT ACTUALLY DOES

- The best evidence in support of VSL #3's digestive health benefit pertains to people with inflammatory bowel conditions, such as ulcerative colitis (UC) and pouchitis.

- Multiple small, randomized controlled trials have found that VSL #3 helped patients with ulcerative colitis achieve remission compared to placebo. It also seems to improve response to standard medications when added as an adjunct therapy. It may also help patients with UC maintain their remission.

- People who have had bowel surgeries and have an ileal pouch also seem to benefit from VSL #3. It helps manage cases of recurrent inflammation of the pouch, called *pouchitis*.

- VSL #3 has been studied as a therapy for people with functional bowel issues, like IBS and constipation, though the results have not been as promising. Two small studies showed no significant improvement in IBS symptoms compared to a placebo among diarrhea-predominant IBS sufferers when taking VSL #3. In a study of thirty patients with constipation, VSL #3 showed promise in terms of improving stool frequency, consistency, and abdominal bloating, though this study was not placebo controlled.

SAFETY AND TOLERANCE CONCERNS

- Like all probiotics, VSL #3 is considered very safe for most everyone except sick infants and immunocompromised people.
- The one exception is among people with a history of SIBO (chapter 8), who are prone to overgrowing even "good" bacteria in their small intestines. VSL #3 and all other bacterial probiotics may "seed" the small bowel and induce a recurrence. Similarly, if you're at high risk for developing SIBO due to having low stomach acid levels from age, an autoimmune disease that decreases stomach acid levels, or use of an acid-reducing medication that ends with -prazole, taking bacterial probiotics may increase this risk.
- VSL #3 is dispensed by pharmacists and should be taken under medical supervision.

DOSING

- VSL #3 is sold in both capsules and powder form. It is available in three dose strengths: 225 billion colony-forming units (CFUs); 450 billion CFUs; and 900 billion CFUs (by prescription only).
- Your doctor will recommend an appropriate dose for your symptoms.

THE BOTTOM LINE?

- Worth a try for patients with constipation if other remedies have not produced satisfactory results. Given its relatively high cost, the need for medical supervision while using it and the still-small amount of evidence supporting its utility, it would not be my first choice as a remedy for constipation.
- (It is my first choice for people with ulcerative colitis and pouchitis, though!)
- Skip it if you have a history of SIBO (chapter 8) or are at high risk for developing SIBO.

Xylose Isomerase (XI)

ALSO MARKETED AS

- Xylosolv

WHAT IT IS

Xylose isomerase (XI) is an enzyme that converts one type of sugar—fructose—into a different type of sugar—glucose. It has been used for decades in the food-processing industry to create high-fructose corn syrup, but more recently has been marketed as a dietary supplement for people with fructose intolerance.

WHAT MARKETERS CLAIM IT DOES

- Prevents gas and bloating from consuming fructose in people with fructose intolerance (malabsorption).

WHAT IT ACTUALLY DOES

- XI converts dietary fructose to glucose in the small intestine. Because glucose is so easy to absorb, this conversion process can prevent the malabsorption-related symptoms related to consuming fructose among people who are fructose intolerant (chapter 9).

- To date, there's been only one study done in humans testing this supplement out, but it happened to be a good-quality one with promising results. In a double-blind, placebo-controlled study of sixty-five people with diagnosed fructose intolerance, those who took xylose isomerase had significantly less nausea and abdominal pain after drinking a fructose-rich drink compared to those given a placebo pill. (There was also less hydrogen gas on their breath, which showed evidence of less bacterial fermentation of the fructose load.) They did not experience less bloating, though.

SAFETY AND TOLERANCE CONCERNS

- XI is generally very safe for most people, with the few exceptions noted below. Since it acts locally in the gut and is not absorbed into the body, the likelihood of side effects from xylose isomerase is minimal.

- It is not suitable for people with a hereditary, metabolic disease called *hereditary fructose intolerance* (*HFI*). If you have HFI, taking XI will not make it safe for you to ingest fructose.

- If you have type 2 diabetes, you should consult your doctor before using xylose isomerase.

DOSING

- For XI to work, you need to take it immediately *before* starting to consume a food or drink that contains fructose. The dose of XI you take must be well matched to the amount of fructose you consume, so test the waters with conservative portions of fructose before going all out.

THE BOTTOM LINE?

- Worth a try for bloating that results from fructose intolerance (chapter 9).

Sources

Listed below are the principal sources I consulted in preparing this book and upon which much of my clinical approach is based. Website URLs are current as of March 2018. Special thanks to Erin Kratzer, MS, RD, for her research support.

In addition to the sources listed below, I referenced the product labels and/or company websites of name-brand medicines and dietary supplements referenced throughout this manuscript for information on dosing, active ingredients, and inactive ingredients. The information cited was current as of May 2017.

Part 2: Upper-Abdominal Bloating That Originates in the Stomach

Barba, E., Burri, E., Accarino, A., Cisternas, D., Quiroga, S., Monclus, E., Navazo, I., Malagelada, J. R., & Azpiroz, F. (2015). Abdominothoracic mechanisms of functional abdominal distension and correction by biofeedback. *Gastroenterology,* *148*(4), 732–739. doi: 10.1053/j.gastro.2014.12.006

Bredenoord, A. J. (2013). Management of belching, hiccups, and aerophagia. *Clinical Gastroenterology and Hepatology, 11*(1), 6–12. doi: 10.1016/j.cgh.2012.09.006

Malagelada, J. R., Accarino, A., & Azpiroz, F. (2013). Bloating and abdominal distension: Old misconceptions and current knowledge. *American Journal of Gastroenterology, 112*(8), 1221–1231. doi: 10.1038/ajg.2017.129

Seeley, R., Stephens, T., & Tate, P. (2006). *Essentials of Anatomy & Physiology* (6th ed.). New York, NY: McGraw-Hill.

Stanghellini, V., Chan, F. K. L., Hasler, W. L., Malagelada, J. R., Suzuki, H., Tack, J., & Talley, N. J. (2016). Gastroduodenal disorders. *Gastroenterology, 150*(6), 1380–1392. doi: 10.1053/j.gastro.2016.02.011

Villoria, A., Azpiroz, F., Burri, E., Cisternas, D., Soldevilla, A., & Malagelada, J. R. (2011). Abdomino-phrenic dyssynergia in patients with abdominal bloating and distension. *American Journal of Gastroenterology, 106*(5), 815–819. doi: 10.1038/ajg.2010.408

Part 3: Lower-Abdominal Bloating That Originates in the Intestines

Biesiekierski, J., Peters, S., Newnham, E., Rosella, O., Muir, J., & Gibson, P. (2013). No effects of gluten in patients with self-reported non-celiac gluten sensitivity after dietary reduction of fermentable, poorly absorbed, short-chain carbohydrates. *Gastroenterology, 145*(2), 320–328. e1-3. doi: 10.1053/j.gastro.2013.04.051

Gibson, P. (2017). The evidence base for efficacy of the low-FODMAP diet in irritable bowel syndrome: Is it ready for prime time as a first-line therapy? *Journal of Gastroenterology and Hepatology, 32*(Suppl 1), 32–35. doi: 10.1111/jgh.13693

Gibson, P., & Shepherd, S. (2010). Evidence-based dietary management of functional gastrointestinal symptoms: The FODMAP approach. *Journal of Gastroenterology and Hepatology, 25*(2), 252–258. doi: 10.1111/j.1440-1746.2009.06149.x

Lacy, B. E., Mearin, F., Chang, L., Chey, W. D., Lembo, A. J., Simren, M., & Spiller, R. (2016). Bowel disorders. *Gastroenterology, 150*(6), 1393–1407. doi: 10.1053/j.gas tro.2016.02.031

Parzanese, I., Qehajaj, D., Patrinicola, F., Aralica, M., Chiriva-Internati, M., Stifter, S., Elli, L., & Grizzi, F. (2017). Celiac disease: From pathophysiology to treatment. *World Journal of Gastrointestinal Pathophysiology, 8*(2), 27–38. doi: 10.4291/wjgp.v8.i2.27

Rao, S., Bharucha, A. E., Chiarioni, G., Felt-Bersma, R., Knowles, C., Malcolm, A., & Wald, A. (2016). Anorectal disorders. *Gastroenterology, 150*(6), 1430–1442. doi: 10.1053/j.gastro.2016.02.009

Rezaie, A., Buresi, M., Lembo, A., Lin, H., McCallum, R., Rao, S., Schmulson, M., Valdovinos, M., Zakko, S., & Pimentel, M. (2017). Hydrogen and methane-based breath testing in gastrointestinal disorders: The North American consensus. *American Journal of Gastroenterology, 112*(5), 775–784. doi: 10.1038/ajg.2017.46

Rezaie, A., Pimentel, M., & Rao, S. (2016). How to test and treat small intestinal bacterial overgrowth: An evidence-based approach. *Current Gastroenterology Reports, 18*(2), 8. doi: 10.1007/s11894-015-0482-9

Seeley, R., Stephens, T., & Tate, P. (2006). *Essentials of Anatomy & Physiology* (6th ed.). New York, NY: McGraw-Hill.

Part 4: Dietary Remedies for Bloating

DATABASES/RAW DATA SOURCES

Department of Agriculture Agricultural Research Service. *USDA Food Composition Databases*. Retrieved from Department of Agriculture website: https://ndb.nal.usda.gov/ndb/.

EBSCO CAM Review Board. Herbs & Supplements: ConsumerLab.com Encyclopedia website. Updated December 15, 2015. Accessed April–May 2017.

Fiber content of foods in common portions. (2004 May). Retrieved from http://huhs.harvard.edu/assets/File/OurServices/Service_Nutrition_Fiber.pdf. As of March 2018, available at https://cookwithkathy.files.wordpress.com/2014/05/sifibre.pdf.

Monash University low FODMAP diet guide. (2018). Retrieved from http://itunes.apple.com.

National Center for Complementary and Integrative Health. Retrieved from National Center for Complementary and Integrative Health website: https://nccih.nih.gov/.

Pennington, J. A. T., & Spungen, J. S. (2009). *Bowes and Church's Food Values of Portions Commonly Used* (19th ed.). Baltimore, MD: Lippincott Williams & Wilkins.

University of Maryland Medical Center. *Complementary and Alternative Medicine Guide*. Retrieved from University of Maryland Medical Center website: https://www.umm.edu/health/medical/altmed.

RESEARCH STUDIES AND SCIENTIFIC REVIEWS

Akobeng, A. K., Elawad, M., & Gordon, M. (2016). Glutamine for induction of remission in Crohn's disease. *Cochrane Database of Systematic Reviews, 2*:CD007348. doi: 10.1002/14651858.CD007348.pub2

Alam, M. S., Roy, P. K., Miah, A. R., Mollick, S. H., Khan, M. R., Mahmud, M. C., & Khatun, S. (2013). Efficacy of peppermint oil in diarrhea predominant IBS—a double-blind randomized placebo-controlled study. *Mymensingh Medical Journal, 22*(1), 27–30.

Aydin, A., Ersöz, G., Tekesin, O., Akçiçek, E., & Tuncyürek, M. (2000). Garlic oil and Helicobacter pylori infection [letter]. *American Journal of Gastroenterology, 95*(2), 563–564.

Betz, O., Kranke, P., Geldner, G., Wulf, H., & Eberhart, L. H. (2005). Is ginger a clinically relevant antiemetic? A systematic review of randomized controlled trials. *Forsch Komplementarmed Klass Naturheilkd, 12*, 14–23.

Boone, S. A., & Shields, K. M. (2005). Treating pregnancy-related nausea and vomiting with ginger. *Annals of Pharmacotherapy, 39*(10), 1710–1713.

Borrelli, F., Capasso, R., Aviello, G., Pittler, M. H., & Izzo, A. A. (2005). Effectiveness and safety of ginger in the treatment of pregnancy-induced nausea and vomiting. *Obstetrics & Gynecology, 105*(4), 849–856.

Brandt, L. J. (2009). An evidence-based position statement on the management of irritable bowel syndrome. *American Journal of Gastroenterology, 104*(Suppl 1), S1–S35. doi: 10.1038/ajg.2008.122

Bunch, T. R., Bond, C., Buhl, K., & Stone, D. (2013). Diatomaceous earth general fact sheet. National Pest Information Center, Oregon State University Extension Services. http://npic.orst.edu/factsheets/degen.html

Casella, S., Leonardi, M., Melai, B., Fratini, F., & Pistelli, L. (2013). The role of diallyl sulfides and dipropyl sulfides in the in vitro antimicrobial activity of the essential oils of garlic, Allium sativum L., and leek, Allium porrum L. *Phytotherapy Research, 27*(3), 380–383. doi: 10.1002/ptr.4725

Cash, B. D., Epstein, M. S., & Shah, S. M. (2016). A novel delivery system of peppermint oil is an effective therapy for irritable bowel syndrome. *Digestive Disease and Sciences, 61*(2), 560–571. doi: 10.1007/s10620-015-3858-7

Chaiyakunapruk, N., Kitikannakorn, N., Nathisuwan, S., Leeprakobboon, K., & Leelasettagool, C. (2006). The efficacy of ginger for the prevention of postoperative nausea and vomiting: A meta-analysis. *American Journal of Obstetrics & Gynecology, 194*(1), 95–99.

Chen, C., Lu, M., Pan, Q., Fichna, J., Zheng, L., Wang, K., Yu, Z., Li, Y., Li, K., Song, A., Liu, Z., Song, Z., & Kreis, M. (2015). Berberine improves intestinal motility and visceral pain in the mouse models mimicking diarrhea-predominant irritable bowel syndrome (IBS-D) symptoms in an opioid-receptor dependent manner. *PLoS ONE, 10*(12), e0145556. doi: 10.1371/journal.pone.0145556

Chen, C., Tao, C., Liu, Z., Lu, M., Pan, Q., Zheng, L., Li, Q., Song, Z., & Fichna, J. (2015). A randomized clinical trial of berberine hydrochloride in patients with diarrhea-predominant irritable bowel syndrome. *Phytotherapy Research, 29*(11), 1822–1827. doi: 10.1002/ptr.5475

Coon, J. T., & Ernst, E. (2002). Systematic review: Herbal medicinal products for non-ulcer dyspepsia. *Alimentary Pharmacology & Therapeutics, 16*:1689–1699.

Currò, D., Ianiro, G., Pecere, S., Bibbò, S., & Cammarota, G. (2017). Probiotics, fibre, and herbal medicinal products for functional and inflammatory bowel disorders. *British Journal of Pharmacology, 174*(11), 1426–1449. doi: 10.1111/bph.13632

Daferera, D. J., Ziogas, B. N., & Polissiou, M. G. (2000). GC-MS analysis of essential oils from some Greek aromatic plants and their fungitoxicity on Penicillium digitatum. *Journal of Agricultural & Food Chemistry, 48*(6), 2576–2581.

Davis, K., Philpott, S., Kumar, D., & Mendal, M. (2006). Randomised double-blind placebo-controlled trial of aloe vera for irritable bowel syndrome. *International Journal of Clinical Practice, 60*(9), 1080–1086.

Di Nardo, G., Oliva, S., Ferrari, F., Mallardo, S., Barbara, G., Cremon, C., Aloi, M., & Cucchiara, S. (2013). Efficacy and tolerability of a-galactosidase in treating gas-related symptoms in children: A randomized, double-blind, placebo-controlled trial. *BMC Gastroenterology, 13*, 142. doi: 10.1186/1347-230X-13-142

Di Stefano, M., Miceli, E., Gotti, S., Missanelli, A., Mazzocchi, S., & Corazza, G. R. (2007). The effects of oral alpha-galactosidase on intestinal gas production and gas-related symptoms. *Digestive Disease and Sciences, 52*(1), 78–83.

Dorman, H. J., & Deans, S. G. (2000). Antimicrobial agents from plants: Antibacterial activity of plant volatile oils. *Journal of Applied Microbiology, 88*(2), 308–316.

Engqvist, A., von Feilitzen, F., Pyk, E., & Reichard, H. (1973). Double-blind trial of deglycyrrhizinated liquorice in gastric ulcer. *Gut, 14*(9), 711–715.

Fleming, V., & Wade, W. E. (2010). A review of laxative therapies for treatment of chronic constipation in older adults. *American Journal of Geriatric Pharmacotherapy, 8*(6), 514–550.

Ford, A. C., Quigley, E. M., Lacy, B. E., Lembo, A. J., Saito, Y. A., Schiller, L. R., Soffer, E. E., Spiegel, B. M., & Moayyedi, P. (2014). Efficacy of prebiotics, probiotics, and synbiotics in irritable bowel syndrome and chronic idiopathic constipation: Systematic review and meta-analysis. *American Journal of Gastroenterology, 109*(10), 1547–1561. doi: 10.1038/ajg.2014.202

Ganiats, T. G., Norcross, W. A., Halverson, A. L., Buford, P. A., & Palinkas, L. A. (1994). Does Beano prevent gas? A double-blind crossover study of oral alpha-galactosidase to treat dietary oligosaccharide intolerance. *Journal of Family Practice, 39*(5), 441–445.

Gao, K. P., Mitsui, T., Fujiki, K., Ishiguro, H., & Kondo, T. (2002). Effects of lactase preparations in asymptomatic individuals with lactase deficiency—gastric digestion of lactose and breath hydrogen analysis. *International Journal of Medical Sciences, 65*(1–2), 21–28.

Gibson, P. R., Newnham, E., Barrett, J. S., Shepherd, S. J., & Muir, J. G. (2007). Review article: Fructose malabsorption and the bigger picture. *Alimentary Pharmacology & Therapeutics, 25*(4), 349–363.

Goldenberg, J. Z., Lytvyn, L., Steurich, J., Parkin, P., Mahant, S., & Johnston, B. C. (2015). Probiotics for the prevention of pediatric antibiotic-associated diarrhea. *Cochrane Database of Systematic Reviews, 12*, CD004827. doi: 10.1002/14651858.CD00 4827.pub4

Grundmann, O., & Yoon, S. L. (2014). Complementary and alternative medicines in irritable bowel syndrome: An integrative view. *World Journal of Gastroenterology, 20*(2), 346–362. doi: 10.3748/wjg.v20.i2.346

Guo, X., & Mei, N. (2016). Aloe vera: A review of toxicity and adverse clinical effects. *Journal of Environmental Science and Health Part C Environmental Carcinogenic Ecotoxicology Reviews, 34*(2), 77–96. doi: 10.1080/10590501.2016.1166826

Habtemariam, S. (2016). Berberine and inflammatory bowel disease: A concise review. *Pharmacology Research, 113*(Pt A), 592–599.

Hale, L. P., Greer, P. K., Trinh, C. T., & Gottfried, M. R. (2005). Treatment with oral bromelain decreases colonic inflammation in the IL-10-decifient murine model of inflammatory bowel disease. *Clinical Immunology, 116*(2), 135–142.

Hall, R. G., Thompson, H., & Strother, A. (1981). Effects of orally administered activated charcoal on intestinal gas. *American Journal of Gastroenterology, 75*(3), 192–196.

Holtmann, G., Haag, S., Adam, B., Funk, P., Wieland, V., & Heydenreich, C. J. (2003). Effects of a fixed combination of peppermint oil and caraway oil on symptoms and quality of life in patients suffering from functional dyspepsia. *Phytomedicine, 10*(Suppl 4), 56–57.

Hunter, J. O., Tuffnell, Q., & Lee, A. J. (1999). Controlled trial of oligofructose in the management of irritable bowel syndrome. *Journal of Nutrition, 129*(Suppl 7), 1451S–1453S.

Jain, N. K., Patel, V. P., & Pitchumoni, C. S. (1986). Efficacy of activated charcoal in reducing intestinal gas: A double-blind clinical trial. *American Journal of Gastroenterology, 81*(7), 532–535.

Kane, S., & Goldberg, M. J. (2000). Letter: Use of bromelain for mild ulcerative colitis. *Annals of Internal Medicine, 132*(8), 680.

Khanna, R., MacDonald, J. K., & Levesque, B. G. (2014). Peppermint oil for the treatment of irritable bowel syndrome: A systematic review and meta-analysis. *Journal of Clinical Gastroenterology, 48*(6), 505–512. doi: 10.1097/MCG.0b013e3182a88357

Ki Cha, B., Mun Jung, S., Hwan Choi, C., Song, I. D., Woong Lee, H., Joon Kim, H., Hyuk, J., Kyung Chang, S., Kim, K., Chung, W. S., & Seo, J. G. (2012). The effect of a multispecies probiotic on the symptoms and fecal microbiota in diarrhea-dominant irritable bowel syndrome: A randomized, double-blind, placebo-controlled trial. *Journal of Clinical Gastroenterology, 46*(3), 220–227. doi: 10.1097/MCG.0b013e31823712b1

Kim, H. J., Camilleri, M., McKinzie, S., Lempke, M. B., Burton, D. D., Thomforde, G. M., & Zinsmeister, A. R. (2003). A randomized controlled trial of a probiotic, VSL#3, on gut transit and symptoms in diarrhoea-predominant irritable bowel syndrome. *Alimentary Pharmacology & Therapeutics, 17*(7), 895–904.

Kim, S. E, Choi, S. C., Park, K. S., Park, M. I., Shin, J. E., Lee, T. H., Jung, K. W., Koo, H. S., & Myung, S. J. (Constipation Research group of Korean Society of Neurogastroenterology and Motility). (2015). Change of Fecal Flora and Effectiveness of the Short-term VSL#3 Probiotic Treatment in Patients with Functional Constipation. *Journal of Neurogastroenterology and Motility, 21*(1), 111–120. doi: 10.5056/jnm14048

Kinnunen, O., & Salokannel, J. (1987). Constipation in elderly long-stay patients: Its treatment by magnesium hydroxide and bulk laxative. *Annals of Clinical Research, 19*(5), 321–323.

Komericki, P., Akkilic-Materna, M., Strimitzer, T., Weyermair, K., Hammer, H. F., & Aberer, W. (2012). Oral xylose isomerages decreases breath hydrogen excretion and improves gastrointestinal symptoms in fructose malabsorption—a double-blind, placebo-controlled study. *Alimentary Pharmacology & Therapeutics, 36*(10), 980–987. doi:10.1111/apt.12057

Lambeau, K. V., & McRorie, J. W., Jr. (2017). Fiber supplements and clinically proven health benefits: How to recognize and recommend an effective fiber therapy. *Journal of the American Association of Nurse Practitioners, 29*(4), 216–223. doi:10.1002/2327-6924.12447

Lambert, R. J., Skandamis, P. N., Coote, P. J., & Nychas, G. J. (2001). A study of the minimum inhibitory concentration and mode of action of oregano essential oil, thymol and carvacrol. *Journal of Applied Microbiology, 91*(3), 453–462.

Lettieri, J., & Bradley, D. (1998). Effects of Beano on the tolerability and pharmacodynamics of acarbose. *Clinical Therapeutics, 20*(3), 497–504.

Levine, B., & Weisman, S. (2004). Enzyme replacement as an effective treatment for the common symptoms of complex carbohydrate intolerance. *Nutrition in Clinical Care, 7*(2), 75–81.

Levine, M. E., Koch, S. Y., & Koch, K. L. (2015). Lipase supplementation before a high-fat meal reduces perceptions of fullness in healthy subjects. *Gut and Liver, 9*(4), 464–469. doi: 10.5009/gnl14005

Lin, M. Y., Dipalma, J. A., Martini, M. C., Gross, C. J., Harlander, S. K., & Savaiano, D. A. (1993). Comparative effects of exogenous lactase (beta-galactosidase) in preparations on in vivo lactose digestion. *Digestive Disease and Sciences, 38*(11), 2022–2027.

Linetzky Waitzbergm, D., Alves Pereira, C. C., Logullo, L., Manzoni Jacintho, T., Almeida, D., Teixeira da Silva, M. L., & Matos de Miranda Torrinhas, R. S. (2012). Microbiota benefits after inulin and partially hydrolized guar gum supplementation: A randomized clinical trial in constipated women. *Nutricion Hospitalaria, 27*(1), 123–129.

Liu, L. W. C. (2011). Chronic constipation: Current treatment options. *Canadian Journal of Gastroenterology, 25*(Suppl B), 22B–28B.

Madisch, A., Heydenreich, C. J., Wieland, V., Hufnagel, R., & Hotz, J. (1999). Treatment of functional dyspepsia with a fixed peppermint oil and caraway oil combination preparation as compared to cisapride. A multicenter, reference-controlled double-blind equivalence study. *Arzneimittelforschung, 49*(11), 925–932.

Madisch, A., Holtmann, G., Plein, K., & Hotz, J. (2004). Treatment of irritable bowel syndrome with herbal preparations: Results of a double-blind, randomized, placebo-controlled, multi-centre trial. *Alimentary Pharmacology & Therapeutics, 19*(3), 271–279.

Malfertheiner, P., & Domínguez-Muñoz, J. E. (1993). Effect of exogenous pancreatic enzymes on gastrointestinal and pancreatic hormone release and gastrointestinal motility. *Digestion, 54*(Suppl 2), 15–20.

Maton, P. N., & Burton, M. E. (1999). Antacids revisited: A review of their clinical pharmacology and recommended therapeutic use. *Drugs, 57*(6), 855–870.

May, B., Köhler, S., & Schneider, B. (2000). Efficacy and tolerability of a fixed combination of peppermint oil and caraway oil in patients suffering from functional dyspepsia. *Alimentary Pharmacology & Therapeutics, 14*(12), 1671–1677.

McRorie, J. W., Jr. (2015). Evidence-based approach to fiber supplements and clinically meaningful health benefits, part 1. *Nutrition Today, 50*(2), 82–89.

McRorie, J. W., Jr. (2015). Evidence-based approach to fiber supplements and clinically meaningful health benefits, part 2. *Nutrition Today, 50*(2), 90–97.

Millea, P. J. (2009). N-acetylcysteine: Multiple clinical applications. *American Family Physician, 80*(3), 265–269.

Montalto, M., Curigliano, V., Santoro, L., Vastola, M., Cammartoa, G., Manna, R., Gasbarrini, A., & Gasbarrini, G. (2006). Management and treatment of lactose malabsorption. *World Journal of Gastroenterology, 12*(2), 187–191.

Moshfegh, A., Friday, J., Goldman, J., Chug-Ahuja, J. (1999). Presence of inulin and oligofructose in the diets of Americans. *The Journal of Nutrition, 129*(7), 1407(S)–1411(S).

Mounsey, A., Raleigh, M., & Wilson, A. (2015). Management of constipation in older adults. *American Family Physician, 92*(6), 500–504.

Mueller-Lissner, S. A., & Wald, A. (2010). Constipation in adults. *BMJ Clinical Evidence, 413.*

Musso, C. G. (2009). Magnesium metabolism in health and disease. *International Urology and Nephrology, 41*(2), 357–362.

National Institutes of Health Office of Dietary Supplements. (2016). Magnesium: Fact sheet for health professionals. Retrieved on National Institute of Health website: https://ods.od.nih.gov/factsheets/Magnesium-HealthProfessional/

Navarro, V. J., Khan, I., Björnsson, E., Seeff, L. B., Serrano, J., & Hoofnagle, J. H. (2017). Liver injury from herbal and dietary supplements. *Hepatology, 65*(1), 363–373. doi: 10.1002/hep.28813

O'Mahony, L., McCarthy, J., Kelly, P., Hurley, G., Luo, F., Chen, K., O'Sullivan, G. C., Kiely, B., Collins, J. K., Shanahan, F., & Quigley, E. M. (2005). Lactobacillus and bifidocaterium in irritable bowel syndrome: Symptom responses and relationship to cytokine profiles. *Gastroenterology, 128*(3), 541–551.

Ottillinger, B., Storr, M., Malfertheiner, P., & Allescher, H. D. (2013). STW 5 (Iberogast)—a safe and effective standard in the treatment of functional gastrointestinal disorders. *Wien Med Wochenschr, 163*(3–4), 65–72.

Pace, F., Pace, M., & Quartarone, G. (2015). Probiotics in digestive diseases: Focus on Lactobacillus GG. *Minerva Gastroenterolical e Dietologica, 61*(4), 273–292.

Pappas, P. G., Kauffman, C. A., Andes, D. R., Clancy, C. J., Marr, K. A., Ostrosky-Zeichner, L., Reboli, A. C., Schuster, M. G., Vazquez, J. A., Walsh, T. J., Zaoutis, T. E., & Sobel, J. D. (2016). Clinical practice guideline for the management of candidiasis: 2016 update by the infectious disease society of America. *Clinical Infectious Diseases, 62*(4), 409–417. doi: 10.1093/cid/civ933

Pare, P., Bridges, R., Champion, M. C., Ganguli, S. C., Gray, J. R., Irvine, E. J., Plourde, V., Poitras, P., Turnbull, G. K., Moayyedi, P., Flook, N., & Collins, S. M. (2007). Recommendations on chronic constipation (including constipation associated with irritable bowel syndrome) treatment. *Canadian Journal of Gastroenterology, 21*(Suppl B), 3B–22B.

Park, S. Y., & Rew, J. S. (2015). Is lipase supplementation before a high-fat meal helpful to patients with functional dyspepsia? *Gut & Liver, 9*(4), 433–434. doi: 10.5009/gnl15206

Portalatinm, M., & Winstead, N. (2012). Medical management of constipation. *Clinics in Colon & Rectal Surgery, 25*(1), 12–19.

Potter, T., Ellis, C., & Levitt, M. (1985). Activated charcoal: In vivo and in vitro studies of effect on gas formation. *Gastroenterology, 88*(3), 620–624.

Ringel-Kulka, T., McRorire, J., & Ringel, Y. (2017). Multi-center, double-blind, randomized, placebo-controlled, parallel-group study to evaluate the benefit of the probiotic Bifidobacterium infantis 35624 in non-patients with symptoms of abdominal discomfort and bloating. *American Journal of Gastroenterology, 112*(1), 145–151. doi: 10.1038/ajg.2016.511

Robinson, M., Rodriguez-Stanley, S., Miner, P. B., McGuire, A. J., Fung, K., & Ciociola, A. A. (2002). Effects of antacid formulation on postprandial oesophageal acidity in patients with a history of episodic heartburn. *Alimentary Pharmacology & Therapeutics, 16*(3), 435–443.

Sakkas, H., & Papadopoulou, C. (2017). Antimicrobial activity of basil, oregano, and thyme essential oils. *Journal of Microbial Biotechnology, 27*(3), 429–438. doi: 10.4014/jmb.1608.08024

Sanders, S. W., Tolmac, K. G., & Reitberg, D. P. (1992). Effect of a single dose of lactase on symptoms and expired hydrogen after lactose challenge in lactose-intolerant subjects. *Journal of Clinical Pharmacology, 11*(6), 533–538.

Silk, D. B., Davis, A., Vulevic, J., Tzortzis, G., & Gibson, G. R. (2009). Clinical trial: The effects of a trans-galactosoligosaccharide prebiotic on faecal microbiota and symptoms of irritable bowel syndrome. *Alimentary Pharmacology & Therapeutics, 29*(5), 508–518.

Slavin, J. (2013). Fiber and prebiotics: Mechanisms and health benefits. *Nutrients, 5*(4), 1417–1437.

Stewart, J. J., Wood, M. J., Wood, C. D., & Mims, M. E. (1991). Effects of ginger on motion sickness susceptibility and gastric function. *Pharmacology, 42*(2), 111–120.

Suarez, F., Levitt, M. D., Adshead, J., & Barkin, J. S. (1999). Pancreatic supplements reduce symptomatic response of healthy subjects to a high-fat meal. *Digestive Disease Science, 44*(7), 1317–1321.

von Arnim, U., Peitz, U., Vinson, B., Gundermann, K. J., & Malfertheiner, P. (2007). STW 5, a phytopharmacon for patients with functional dyspepsia: Results of a multicenter, placebo-controlled double-blind study. *American Journal of Gastroenterology, 102*(6), 1268–1275.

White, B. (2007). Ginger: An overview. *American Family Physician, 75*(11), 1689–1691.

Whorwell, P. J., Altringer, L., Morel, J., Bond, Y., Charbonneau, D., O'Mahony, L., Kiely, B., Shanahan, F., & Quigley, E. M. (2006). Efficacy of an encapsulated probiotic Bifidobacterium infantis 35624 in women with irritable bowel syndrome. *American Journal of Gastroenterology, 101*(7), 1581–1590.

Index

aloe vera (aloe barbadensis), 256–57
alpha-galactosidase, 128, 129, 203, 257–58
amylases, 119
Ananas comosus (pineapple) extract
(bromelain), 129, 261–62
anatomy, 12–14
Anna Karenina (Tolstoy), 5
anorectal manometry, 39–40, 85
antacids, 46, 48–49, 51, 57, 61
antianxiety medications, 72
antibiotics
probiotics and, 114, 115
prokinetic properties in, 28–29
SIBO (small intestinal bacterial
overgrowth) and, 103, 108–10, 114
antidepressants, 62
antiemetics, 29
antispasmodic medications, 72
anxiety, 38, 71, 81
medications for, 72
anus, 14, 80
APD, *see* abdomino-phrenic dyssynergia
appetite, 25, 26
Apple-Peach Crumble for Two, 196
Artichoke and White Bean Flatbreads,
184
ascorbic acid (vitamin C), 297–98
Asparagus and Rice Soup, 178
avocado
Avocado Cilantro Toasts with
Scrambled Egg Whites, 172
Grilled Fish and Zucchini Tacos with
Mango-Avocado Salsa, 186–87

bacteria
in colon, 90, 96, 101, 102, 109, 118–22
"good" and "bad," 102
in small intestine, overgrowth of,
see small intestinal bacterial
overgrowth
baking soda, 48–49
Banana-Chocolate Mousse, 198
basil
Pesto Pasta with Salmon and Green
Beans, 232–33
Zucchini with Pesto, 242
Beano, Bean-zyme, Beanaid (alpha-
galactosidase), 128, 129, 203, 257–58
beans, 129, 143, 152
gas and, 128, 167–68

Vegetarian Couscous, 189–90
White Bean and Artichoke
Flatbreads, 184
beef
Mexican Beef Bowl, 226–27
Thai Beef Salad, 220–21
behavioral therapy, 72
Benefiber (soluble-fiber supplements),
159, 295–97
berberine (*Berberis aristanta, B. petiolaris,
B. vulgaris, B. darwinii*), 259–60
berries
Get Your Greens Smoothie, 175
Meringue Nests with Lime Curd and
Berries, 244–46
betaine HCl (betaine hydrochloride),
260–61
bezoars, 28, 33–34
Bifidobacteria, 254, 298–99
bile, 103
bile acid malabsorption, 103
binge eating, 42–43
biofeedback, 41, 92–93
bismuth subsalicylate, 49
Bloated Belly Whisperer Quiz, 10,
14–20
bloating, 3–9
dietary remedies for, *see* diet
lower-abdominal, originating in the
intestines, 77–148; *see also*
carbohydrate intolerances; celiac
disease; constipation; pancreatic
insufficiency; small intestinal
bacterial overgrowth
upper-abdominal, originating in
stomach, 21–75; *see also*
abdomino-phrenic dyssynergia;
aerophagia; classic indigestion;
functional dyspepsia; gastroparesis
blood sugar, 25
high (hyperglycemia), 24, 33
low (hypoglycemia), 105
blood tests, 48, 107, 125
for celiac disease, 141, 142
Bon Appétit, 8
botulinum toxin (Botox), 93
Bravo test, 59–60
breakfast, GI Gentle
Avocado Cilantro Toasts with
Scrambled Egg Whites, 172

chicken (*continued*)

Greek-Style Braised Chicken Thighs with Olives and Red Bell Peppers, 187–88

Low-FODMAP Broth, 222–23

Chili-Lime Chicken with Cilantro-Cumin Rice, 234–35

chlorogenic acid, 96

chocolate

Chocolate-Banana Mousse, 198

Coconut-Walnut Brownies, 243–44

Peanut Butter-Chocolate Chip Oatmeal Cookies, 246–47

Chooz (calcium carbonate), 48, 51, 57, 262–63

cilantro

Avocado Cilantro Toasts with Scrambled Egg Whites, 172

Chili-Lime Chicken with Cilantro-Cumin Rice, 234–35

Cinnamon Syrup, Citrus Salad with, 242–43

Citrucel (soluble-fiber supplements), 159, 295–97

Citrus Salad with Cinnamon Syrup, 242–43

classic indigestion, 45–54, 157

bloating from, 46–47

causes of, 46

diagnosing, 47–48

dietary treatment for, 50–54

gluten-free diet and, 143

medical treatment for, 48–50

treating, 48–54

coconut

Coconut-Walnut Brownies, 243–44

Pumpkin Seed Coconut Granola (Nut-Free), 215

coffee, 96

cognitive behavioral therapy (CBT), 72

colectomy, 91

colitis, 112

colon (large intestine), 6, 14, 79–80, 101

bacteria in, 90, 96, 101, 102, 109, 118–22

blockage of, 84

surgery to remove, 91

colonic inertia, 89, 90

colonic treatments (colon hydrotherapy), 90

colonoscopy, 107–8

condiments, 208–9

constipation, 18, 79–100

APD (abdomino-phrenic dyssynergia) and, 17–18

bloating from, 82–83

case history of, 97–100

causes of, 80–81

cycle of, 82

diagnosing, 83–86

dietary treatments for, 93–100

gastroparesis and, 17

gluten-free diet and, 143

IBS-related, 80, 86–91, 158, 159, 160

medical treatments for, 86–93

opioid-induced, 80, 160

from pelvic floor dysfunction, 80–81, 91–93, 158, 159

SIBO (small intestinal bacterial overgrowth) and, 104–5

slow-transit, 80, 86–91, 154, 158, 159

and step stool for squatting, 92

surgery for, 91

symptoms and types of, 80, 81

treating, 86–100

cookies

Low-Fat Pumpkin Spice Pillow Cookies, 198–99

Peanut Butter-Chocolate Chip Oatmeal Cookies, 246–47

corn

Corn and Scallop Chowder, 224–25

Mexican Beef Bowl, 226–27

cortisol, 96

Couscous, Vegetarian, 189–90

CPAP machines, 70, 71

Crohn's disease, 103, 105, 112, 200

cucumbers

Cucumber and Melon Salad, 177

Green Onion Tzatziki, 188–89

Hawaiian-Style Tuna Poke Bowl, 180–81

Mexican Beef Bowl, 226–27

Thai Beef Salad, 220–21

Culturelle probiotic, 263–65

Cumin-Cilantro Rice, Chili-Lime Chicken with, 234–35

tofu
  Moroccan-Flavored Tofu Stew over
    Quinoa, 230–31
  Mushroom Tofu Scramble, 174
  Southeast Asian-Flavored Baked Tofu
    with Shiitakes, 190–91
Tolstoy, Leo, 5
tomatoes
  Asian Niçoise-Style Salad, 219–20
  Chicken Tortilla Soup, 223–24
  Creamy Polenta with Ratatouille,
    217–18
  Mexican Beef Bowl, 226–27
  Moroccan-Flavored Tofu Stew over
    Quinoa, 230–31
tortillas
  Chicken Tortilla Soup, 223–24
  Grilled Fish and Zucchini Tacos with
    Mango-Avocado Salsa, 186–87
transenteric studies, 27, 84–85
trauma, 38, 81
tricyclic antidepressants (TCAs), 62
TUMS (calcium carbonate), 48, 51, 57,
    262–63
tuna
  Asian Niçoise-Style Salad, 219–20
  Grilled Fish and Zucchini Tacos with
    Mango-Avocado Salsa, 186–87
  Hawaiian-Style Tuna Poke Bowl,
    180–81
turkey
  Tarragon and Mustard Turkey
    Burgers, 236–37
  Turkey, Bell Pepper, and Sweet Potato
    Hash, 185–86
Tzatziki, Green Onion, 188–89

ulcers, 58
upper-GI series, 27

vegetables
  in allium family, 205–6
  in GI Gentle diet, 163–65
  in low-FODMAP diet, 205–6
vegetable side dishes, GI Gentle
  Butternut Squash Spoonbread, 191–92
  Moroccan Spiced Carrots, 194

Pub-Style Smashed Peas with Mint,
    192–93
  Roasted Cauliflower "Steaks," 193–94
vegetable side dishes, low-FODMAP
  Green Beans with Pecans, 241
  Herb-Roasted Vegetables, 240–41
  Roasted Kabocha Squash with Sage,
    238–39
  Zucchini with Pesto, 242
vitamins
  A, D, E, and K, 138
  B_{12}, 105
  C, 297–98
  deficiencies of, 103, 105
  fat soluble, 138
  water soluble, 138, 297
vomiting, 25, 47

Walnut-Coconut Brownies, 243–44
weight
  fiber and, 152
  gastroparesis and, 25–26
wheat, 111, 127, 144, 201, 206
  gluten in, see gluten

X-rays, 83–84
xylitol, 121, 202
xylose isomerase (XI; Xylosolv), 128,
    203, 299–300

yogurt
  Green Onion Tzatziki, 188–89
  Mexican Beef Bowl, 226–27
  Salmon Cakes with Mustard-Dill-
    Yogurt Sauce and Riced
    Cauliflower, 182–83

Zingiber officinale (ginger) extracts and
    teas, 274–75
zucchini
  Creamy Polenta with Ratatouille,
    217–18
  Grilled Fish and Zucchini Tacos with
    Mango-Avocado Salsa, 186–87
  Mexican Beef Bowl, 226–27
  Vegetarian Couscous, 189–90
  Zucchini with Pesto, 242